Schopenhauer and Adorno on Bodily Suffering

Schopenhauer and Adorno on Bodily Suffering

A Comparative Analysis

Mathijs Peters
'Postwachstumskolleg', Friedrich Schiller University of Jena, Germany

palgrave
macmillan

First published 2014 by
PALGRAVE MACMILLAN

Palgrave Macmillan in the UK is an imprint of Macmillan Publishers Limited, registered in England, company number 785998, of Houndmills, Basingstoke, Hampshire RG21 6XS.

Palgrave Macmillan in the US is a division of St Martin's Press LLC, 175 Fifth Avenue, New York, NY 10010.

Palgrave Macmillan is the global academic imprint of the above companies and has companies and representatives throughout the world.

Palgrave® and Macmillan® are registered trademarks in the United States, the United Kingdom, Europe and other countries

ISBN: 978–1–137–41216–4

This book is printed on paper suitable for recycling and made from fully managed and sustained forest sources. Logging, pulping and manufacturing processes are expected to conform to the environmental regulations of the country of origin.

A catalogue record for this book is available from the British Library.

Library of Congress Cataloging-in-Publication Data

Peters, Mathijs, 1982–
Schopenhauer and Adorno on bodily suffering : a comparative analysis / Mathijs Peters, independent scholar, the Netherlands.
pages cm
Includes bibliographical references and index.
ISBN 978–1–137–41216–4
1. Suffering. 2. Pain. 3. Schopenhauer, Arthur, 1788–1860. 4. Adorno, Theodor W., 1903–1969. I. Title.

B105.S79P48 2014
128′.4—dc23 2014029420

Transferred to Digital Printing in 2014

To my parents, Adri and Hanneke
In memory of Mohammed Kader Majid

Contents

Preface

My interest in the themes I discuss in this study was sparked when I first read Adorno's interpretation of Homer's *Odyssey* in *Dialectic of Enlightenment*. Never before had I read such a fascinating text, which not only develops a radical critique of modernity, but also radiates with passion for philosophy, literature, history, sociology and psychoanalysis and does this in a unique form. I recognized a similar passion in the beautifully written works of Schopenhauer, in whom I initially became interested through Nietzsche and Gerard Reve, but to whose reflections on corporeal suffering and bodily compassion I later returned when I discovered similar themes in the writings of Marx, Adorno, Foucault and Merleau-Ponty.

I became especially fascinated by the peculiar mixture of pessimism and optimism that characterizes the works of both Schopenhauer and Adorno. They are convinced that the world we live in and the social and cultural conditions that structure our lives and that we have shaped ourselves are not necessarily good, and I agree with them: the existence of phenomena as diverse as extreme hunger, war, genocide, chemical weapons, human trafficking, institutionalized inequality, racism, discrimination, sexism, xenophobia and homophobia makes it impossible to claim otherwise. But their pessimism is entwined with a hopeful emphasis on the attempt to eradicate suffering and to constitute experiences of happiness and peace. The works of both express a vulnerable but powerful focus on the human ability to feel compassion and an inspiring appreciation of the arts, especially of literature and music.

Schopenhauer and Adorno keep asking the following question: what kind of life can be lived in a world like this? And their philosophical attempts to answer this question already express hope, driven by a concern with human and non-human suffering and a longing for happiness and peace. This book might not be very optimistic, but I hope that it expresses a similar entwinement of despair and optimism as I found in the works of Schopenhauer and Adorno.

I first read Adorno's interpretation of the *Odyssey* for Bert van den Brink's course on social and political philosophy at Utrecht University. I owe Bert an enormous debt: not only did he supervise my master's thesis on Nietzsche, Adorno and Foucault, he also encouraged me to spend a year as a visiting student at The New School for Social Research. This was made possible by grants awarded to me by Nuffic (the Netherlands organization for international cooperation in higher education) and the Prins Bernhard Cultuurfonds, for which I am very grateful.

After my stay in New York, I undertook further research at the University of Essex, during which I also spent a year at the Institut Catholique de Paris to study French phenomenology. I want to thank Peter Dews, at the University of Essex, for his help and advice, as well as Béatrice Han-Pile and Christopher Janaway, especially for pressing me on the issue of normativity.

My thanks also go out to those who criticized papers that partly revolved around the issues developed in this book and that I presented at the 4th, 5th and 6th International Critical Theory Conferences at the John Felice Rome Center of Loyola University Chicago, and at the 2012 Philosophy and Social Sciences Colloquium in Prague.

Undertaking this kind of research is not easy and takes its toll on one's well-being. First, I therefore want to thank those of my family who believed in my ability to finish this study and kept supporting me, each in their own way: Hanneke and Adri, Machteld, Marije, Daniel, Nadia, Yara and Isis, Judith, Christiaan, Isaac, Nathan and Rachel, Trees, Chris, Rosa and Vincent, Freek and Barbara.

My thanks furthermore go out to those who prevented me from disappearing into my research, either by pulling me out of my books into the world of the social; by relativizing the endeavour itself; by bombarding me with critical questions; or by providing me with Seagalogical escapism: Roald, Hugo, Thijs, Guido, Joop, Emile, Rogier, Bart and Koen.

I also want to thank the family of Barez for supporting me and my research and for introducing me to a new world: Kaak Mohammed, Sabeha khan, Bakhcha, Sardar and Yaad, Parzijn, Kosar, Laas and Wiena, Shapol, Narine and Nashmile, Shara, Alan and Helana, Twana, Gashbin and Lani, and Dana.

Lastly, I want to thank Barez; it is impossible to put into words how much your love and support means to me.

List of Abbreviations

Works by Adorno

AE	*Against Epistemology: A Metacritique; Studies in Husserl and the Phenomenological Antinomies*, transl. W. Domingo.
AT	*Aesthetic Theory*, transl. R. Hullot-Kentor.
DE	*Dialectic of Enlightenment: Philosophical Fragments* [with Max Horkheimer], transl. E. Jephcott.
EA	'Education after Auschwitz', transl. H.W. Pickford.
HF	*History and Freedom: Lectures 1964–1965*, ed. R. Tiedemann, transl. R. Livingstone.
LND	*Lectures on Negative Dialectics: Fragments of a Lecture Course 1965/1966*, ed. R. Tiedemann, transl. R. Livingstone.
M	*Metaphysics – Concepts and Problems: Lectures 1965*, ed. R. Tiedemann, transl. E. Jephcott.
MM	*Minima Moralia: Reflections from Damaged Life*, transl. E. Jephcott.
ND	*Negative Dialectics*, transl. E.B. Ashton.
NK	'Notes on Kafka', transl. S. Weber, S. Weber Nicholsen.
PMM	*Philosophy of Modern Music*, transl. A.G. Mitchell, W.V. Blomster.
PMP	*Problems of Moral Philosophy: Lectures 1963*, ed. T. Schröder, transl. R. Livingstone.
SO	'On Subject and Object', transl. H.W. Pickford.
UE	'Trying to Understand *Endgame*', transl. S.W. Nicholsen.

Works by Schopenhauer

BM	*On the Basis of Morality*, transl. E.F.J. Payne.
DS	'Additional Remarks on the Doctrine of the Suffering of the World', transl. E.F.J. Payne.
FR	*On the Fourfold Root of the Principle of Sufficient Reason*, transl. Mme. K. Hillebrand.
MS	*Metaphysik der Sitten*, Philosophische Vorlesungen, Teil IV, ed. V. Spierling.
WN	*On the Will in Nature*, transl. Mme. K. Hillebrand.

WWR-I *The World as Will and Representation*, vol. 1, transl. E.F.J. Payne.

WWR-II *The World as Will and Representation*, vol. 2, transl. E.F.J. Payne.

1 Introduction

In the Penal Colony

In his short story *In the Penal Colony*, Franz Kafka describes a torture and execution device that carves the commandment broken by a condemned prisoner into his body, a procedure that takes twelve hours and results in the prisoner's death. The workings of the machine are described in a distant, cold and impersonal way that contrasts acutely with the gruesome suffering undergone by the machine's victim.

The cold and objective style of the story – the 'that's the way it is' that, as Adorno observes in his essay on the author, each sentence written by Kafka underscores[1] – reflects the indifference of the Officer, one of its four characters, who worships the machine and does not display or feel compassion with its victim. He is indifferent to the observation that the tortured prisoner's body is in pain. With all its force, this body fights the pain that engulfs it and with the same force the suffering prisoner fights against the pain that makes him a slave to the materiality of his body; that pulls him into the grim reality of his suffering flesh.

Delighted with the efficient way in which the machine manages to torture its victims to death in one of the most gruesome and at the same time slowest ways possible, the Officer describes its workings as follows:

> The harrow is starting to write, once it's completed the first phase of writing on the man's back, the cotton-wool roll comes down and slowly turns the body on to its side, to offer clean space to the harrow. At the same time, the raw parts already inscribed are pressed against the cotton-wool; its special finish immediately staunches the bleeding, and prepares the surface for a deepening of the writing. The

> jagged edges of the harrow here strip the cotton-wool off the wounds as the body is further rotated, and drop it into the trench, and then the harrow gets to work again. Its script steadily deepens over twelve hours. For the first six of them the condemned man lives almost as before, only he experiences pain. After two hours the felt is taken away, because the man has no strength with which to scream.[2]

The objectification of the machine's victim and of the pain it causes, understood as mere functions of its workings, replaceable parts in a precise and rational calculation, finds its conclusion in the Officer's description of the end of the execution: 'the harrow pierces him through, and tosses him into the pit, where the body smacks down on the bloody water and cotton-wool. That concludes the judgment, and we, the soldier and myself, shovel some earth over him.'[3] The prisoner has been robbed of his individuality, reduced to a suffering object and, eventually, to a worthless thing, garbage.

Kafka's story has been interpreted in different ways. Besides its religious references – the machine's victim is said to undergo a mystical experience once his wounds 'decipher' the rule he has broken, becoming a materialization of the objectivity of the commandment[4] – many have focused on its social and political meanings.[5] Others have argued that the machine's efficiency can be understood as illustrating the Foucaultian idea that the modern subject is constituted by practices of subordination and normalization that are surrounded by an aura of scientific objectivity and that are aimed at the body.[6]

In this book, I want to focus on several related aspects of the human condition that Kafka refers to with objective preciseness: the sheer material existence as flesh that makes every embodied being vulnerable to pain and suffering; the coldness displayed towards the machine's victim; and the responses of the story's readers – more specifically, those of abhorrence and of compassion – that may conflict radically with this coldness. Adorno insightfully describes the bodily feeling of *Unheimlichkeit* that Kafka's stories trigger in their readers as follows:

> Among Kafka's presuppositions, not the least is that the contemplative relation between text and reader is shaken to its very roots. His texts are designed not to sustain a constant distance between themselves and their victim but rather to agitate his feelings to a point where he fears that the narrative will shoot toward him like a locomotive in a three-dimensional film.[7]

In the same essay Adorno argues that, in a radical form, Kafka's stories reflect social, political and cultural structures under which the suffering of living creatures is presented as necessary or approached with indifference; a 'social whole in which those whom society holds in its grip and through whom it maintains itself become superfluous.'[8]

Adorno links these observations to the concentration camps constructed under the National Socialist regime. He thereby mainly focuses on the extreme kind of corporeal suffering that took place in these camps, a kind of suffering that reduces individuals to their bodies, robs them of their particularity and of their ability to live, like the prisoner in Kafka's story who is eventually reduced to a disposable object:

> History becomes hell in Kafka because the chance that might have saved it was missed.... In the concentration camps, the boundary between life and death was eradicated. A middle ground was created, inhabited by living skeletons and putrefying bodies, victims unable to take their own lives, Satan's laughter at the hope of abolishing death. As in Kafka's twisted epics, what perished there was that which had provided the criterion of experience – life lived out to its end.[9]

This passage brings us to philosophy and to the moral drive behind the reflections developed in this book. With the first line of his chief work, *Negative Dialectics*, Adorno links the observation that 'history became hell because the chance that might have saved it was missed' to the role of philosophy: 'Philosophy, which once was obsolete, lives on because the moment to realize it was missed', and argues that philosophy is therefore 'obliged ruthlessly to criticize itself'.[10]

Adorno herewith refers to Marx, who famously claimed in *Theses on Feuerbach* that 'the philosophers have only interpreted the world, in various ways; the point is to change it'.[11] Adorno contrasts this idea with a diagnosis of the actual course of history: he observes that philosophers, in fact, failed to change the world for the better and that enlightenment ideals like rationality, autonomy and freedom culminated in the barbarity of Auschwitz. We therefore have to re-evaluate Marx's idea and the role that philosophy can and should play: the horrors of the world, Adorno argues, the catastrophes that scientific progress and rational thought eventually culminated in, force the philosopher to reflect and to think critically. Pulling the thinking mind down into the world itself, a world characterized, in Adorno's view, by suffering and barbarity, would only make philosophy into an uncritical accomplice of this world, of 'Kafka's hell'.

Adorno mainly refers to Nazi Germany in this context, but also describes the war in Vietnam as proving the continuing existence of 'the world of torture that began with Auschwitz'.[12] Furthermore, we only have to think of horrible recent events as diverse as the Rwandan genocide, the war in Darfur, the Srebrenica massacre, the Al-Anfal Campaign in Iraqi Kurdistan, the torturing in Abu Ghraib Prison, Guantanamo Bay, the Syrian Civil War, the hunger crisis in West Africa, or the scale to which human trafficking has developed today, to realize that several important and promising developments that took place after World War II – technological and scientific progress, the ready availability of more natural resources, the ongoing process of globalization, the modernization of the media – have not necessarily gone hand in hand with a decrease in human suffering.

Following Adorno's emphasis on reflection, this study is driven by the (moral) attempt to critically reflect on bodily suffering, our compassionate responses to this suffering, and the failure of humanity to eradicate suffering. It thereby revolves around several of the questions that arise from Kafka's story and that are emphasized by Adorno's essay on the author: What makes people indifferent to the suffering of others or even willing to inflict pain on them? Why have we not succeeded, given our technological and scientific progress and given the premises and promises of enlightenment thinking, in eradicating unnecessary suffering? And what do these observations mean for our (philosophical) ideas about compassion, rationality, morality, happiness and peace?

Arthur Schopenhauer and Theodor W. Adorno

Similarities

I will address these questions by discussing the manner in which two German philosophers try to answer them: Arthur Schopenhauer (1788–860) and the above-mentioned Theodor W. Adorno (1903–69).

I want to discuss these particular thinkers since, as I aim to show in this book, the observations and problems that arise from a comparison of the two constitute a unique and very critical diagnosis of the human condition that is still relevant today. In the works of few other philosophers does the pain of living beings play such a prominent role as in those of Schopenhauer and Adorno. The works of both revolve, almost obsessively, around the question how people, sharing the same existence as corporeal creatures equally vulnerable to pain and suffering, are able to inflict, actively or passively, experiences on other beings that, if inflicted upon themselves, they would reject with all their might.[13] Both authors thereby directly confront what could be called 'enlightenment optimism', emphasizing the power of rationality, autonomy, self-control, progress and human emancipation, with grim and pessimistic observations of a materialistic and somatic nature, often arising from their sensitivity towards corporeal suffering.[14]

In the works of Schopenhauer, it is mostly slavery – still widespread in his time – that returns as an example of the institutionalized manner in which people are capable of hurting and dehumanizing each other.[15] But he also refers to other kinds of suffering to develop a diagnosis of humanity:

> How man deals with man is seen, for example, in Negro slavery, the ultimate object of which is sugar and coffee. However, we need not go so far; to enter at the age of five a cotton-spinning or other factory, and from then on to sit there every day first ten, then twelve, and finally fourteen hours, and perform the same mechanical work, is to purchase dearly the pressure of drawing breath. But this is the fate of millions, and many more millions have an analogous fate.[16]

As illustrated by the passage from his essay on Kafka cited above, the thought of Adorno is overshadowed by the barbarity to which he refers with the word 'Auschwitz'.

It is no coincidence that Schopenhauer and Adorno both mention the effect that the 1755 earthquake of Lisbon had on Voltaire, who used this disaster in his satirical novella *Candide* to criticize Leibniz's idea that 'this is the best of all possible worlds'.[17] Schopenhauer makes the following ironic observation in *The World as Will and Representation*:

> I cannot assign to ... that methodical and broad development of optimism, ... any other merit than that it later gave rise to the immortal *Candide* of the great Voltaire. In this way, of course, Leibniz's oft-repeated and lame excuse for the vile of the world, namely that the bad sometimes produces the good, obtained proof that for him was unexpected. Even by the name of his hero, Voltaire indicated that it needed only sincerity to recognize the opposite of optimism. Actually optimism cuts so strange a figure on this scene of sin, suffering, and death, that we should be forced to regard it as irony if we did not have an adequate explanation of its origin in its secret source (namely hypocritical flattery with an offensive confidence in its success ...) .... But against the palpably sophistical proofs of Leibniz that this is the

> best of all possible worlds, we may even oppose seriously and honestly the proof that it is the worst of all possible worlds.[18]

And in Adorno's *Negative Dialectics* the following passage can be found, in which the natural disaster that hit Lisbon is compared to the industrialized killing of millions of people in the death camps of Nazi Germany:

> The earthquake of Lisbon sufficed to cure Voltaire of the theodicy of Leibniz, and the visible disaster of the first nature was insignificant in comparison with the second, social one, which defies human imagination as it distils a real hell from human evil.[19]

Whereas Schopenhauer's pessimism is summarized by the claim that 'this world itself is the worst of all possible worlds',[20] Adorno's negative diagnosis of the world finds expression in the phrase 'the whole is the wrong'.[21] Referring to Brecht, furthermore, the latter even describes the culture that came after Auschwitz as 'built of dogshit'.[22]

Differences

With Adorno's reference to a disaster of a second and social nature, we arrive at the most important difference between these two thinkers.[23] Whereas Schopenhauer can be characterized as a metaphysical monist with naturalistic and mystical influences, Adorno is a Hegelian Marxist. As we will see, Schopenhauer's claim that this is the worst of all possible worlds is rooted in observations on the metaphysical kernel of the universe and on the manner in which this kernel manifests itself in the nature of everything that exists in this world, including human beings. This means that the wrongness of the world, in Schopenhauer's view, is not caused by a specific historical situation that may be subject to change, but is rooted in the unchangeable and ahistorical *in-itself* of the universe. Herewith, Schopenhauer does not imply that political or social structures do not cause suffering – his critique of the power hold by religious traditions and of the politically and socially organized practice of slavery are examples of this – but he believes these human-made institutions follow from a deeper-lying and unchangeable human essence.

Adorno's claim that the whole is the wrong, on the other hand – a parody of Hegel's dictum *Das Wahre ist das Ganze* ('the whole is the true' or 'the true is the whole')[24] – forms a deeply historical diagnosis of the social, political, cultural and economic characteristics of the status quo he criticized. Unlike Schopenhauer, who, as we will see, argues that human beings can only find enlightenment and salvation in a mystical turning away from the world as a whole, Adorno leaves the possibility open that the reality he criticizes can be bettered by changing the man-made structures and mechanisms that hold this reality under their spell.[25] Furthermore, since human beings are deeply social creatures and are shaped by social categories, happiness can only be found, in his view, by changing the social conditions under which people live.[26]

We find a (perhaps caricatural) illustration of this difference between these two authors in the USSR's official judgement on Schopenhauer. According to the Soviet ideologists, Schopenhauer's works are reactionary, *kleinbürgerlich*, anti-working class (*arbeiterfeindlich*), decadent and conservative.[27] The Hungarian Marxist philosopher Georg Lukács arrived at a similar conclusion. He famously characterized Schopenhauer's philosophy as follows: 'Schopenhauer's system, well laid-out and architecturally ingenious in form – rises up like a modern luxury hotel on the brink of the abyss, nothingness and futility. And the daily sight of the abyss, between leisurely enjoyment of meals or works of art, can only enhance one's pleasure at this elegant comfort.'[28]

Schopenhauer, in other words, discusses the horrors of the world without being involved in this world itself, reflecting on its barbarity but claiming at the same time that the circumstances that cause human suffering cannot be changed. Furthermore, his theory slides down into irrationalism, Lukács observes – into a celebration of a mystical turning away that completely ignores the possibility of making the world itself into a better place by changing its economic, political, cultural and social realities. Schopenhauer's thought, to summarize Lukács' view, is defined by ahistorical egotism, and we will see that this critique indeed found its way into some of Adorno's most negative references to Schopenhauer.[29]

A second difference between Schopenhauer and Adorno is the influence and continuing relevance of their works. Whereas Adorno achieved academic success and became a well-known public intellectual in Germany, especially during the 1950s and 1960s, Schopenhauer was not very successful during the greatest part of his lifetime.[30] The publication of his chief work *The World as Will and Representation* at the end of 1818, as well as of a largely expanded version of this same work in 1844 went by largely unnoticed. He only achieved fame with the 1851 publication of *Parerga and Paralipomena*, a collection of essays and philosophical reflections of which especially the part *Aphorisms on the Wisdom of Life* became popular and was published as a separate book. However, this fame did not last very long and perhaps Schopenhauer had a more important influence on artists than on academic philosophers – Wagner, Mahler, Richard Strauss, Dvorák, Schönberg, Tolstoy, Turgenev, Zola,

Maupassant, Proust, Hardy, Conrad, Thomas Mann, Gide, Lawrence, Gissing, Huysmans, Borges, Beckett, Thomas, Maeterlinck, Reve and Houellebecq all explicitly or implicitly noted Schopenhauer's influence on their outlook on the world and their ideas on art.[31] Even the show-runner of HBO's hit television series *True Detective* mentions the influence of Schopenhauer's ideas on the show's narrative and themes.[32]

There are many reasons for Schopenhauer's current position in the academic world. We can think of the sometimes highly implausible metaphysical conclusions he arrives at (discussed in Chapter 3), his rather ridiculous misogynistic essay 'On Women',[33] the manner in which some of his own frustrations and depressions too uncritically found their way into his philosophical system, and his *ad hominem* attacks on the 'clumsy and senseless charlatan Hegel',[34] whose thought he defined as characterized by 'shallowness, lack of culture and of knowledge'.[35]

Why a comparative analysis?

The theories of Schopenhauer and Adorno will be comprehensively discussed in this book, but this brief overview of the differences between the two makes it necessary to first answer the question of why I believe that it is fruitful to compare these thinkers *at all*. Indeed, although the influences of authors like Kant, Hegel, Kierkegaard, Marx, Nietzsche, Weber, Husserl, Freud, Lukács and Benjamin on the works of Adorno have been discussed extensively, the possible similarities between Schopenhauer and Adorno have been largely ignored. This is especially the case in the English-speaking academic world and holds true for both studies of Schopenhauer and of Adorno.[36] Telling, perhaps, is the fact that Adorno is mentioned only once in *The Cambridge Companion to Schopenhauer*: in his introduction, Christopher Janaway cites one of Adorno's most negative references to Schopenhauer, which describes him as a 'peevish ancestor of existential philosophy and malicious heir of the great speculators'.[37] The same holds true for the recent *A Companion to Schopenhauer*, in which Bart Vandenabeele lists Adorno as one of the many philosophers who 'totally neglected or dismissed' Schopenhauer.[38]

Praise

Vandenabeele's statement, however, is far too strong, which brings me to my reasons for comparing Schopenhauer and Adorno in this book. My first reason is that Adorno did not 'totally neglect or dismiss' Schopenhauer. As we will see, Adorno often refers to him and praises, for example, the negative nature of Schopenhauer's metaphysics and his sensitivity to the suffering of human and non-human animals, specifically mentioning how these aspects of his thought found their way into a critique of Kant and Hegel. In his lectures on *Negative Dialectics*, for example, Adorno states: 'I believe that it is Schopenhauer's undying achievement, however critical we may be of his philosophy in other respects, that on precisely this issue – that is, the point where he breaks with and destroys the theodicy of suffering – we must say that Schopenhauer has escaped from the ideology of the philosophical tradition.'[39]

Furthermore, Adorno frequently refers to Schopenhauer's ideas on freedom, on subjectivity, on the 'veil of Maya' and especially on the permeation of the world with the *principium individuationis* as expressing a truth moment about the times in which he lived. Even though Adorno may not agree with many of Schopenhauer's ideas, the latter's philosophy is important to him as a reflection of a way of thinking and being. I return to this observation below.

Max Horkheimer

This brings me to a second reason for comparing Schopenhauer and Adorno: the former influenced several authors who were enormously important to the latter. The first of these is Max Horkheimer,[40] Adorno's most important intellectual corroborator and director of the *Institut für Sozialforschung*, the intellectual home of Critical Theory and the *Frankfurter Schule*, to which Adorno belonged. Schopenhauer's abovementioned *Aphorisms on the Wisdom of Life* was the first philosophical book Horkheimer read in his life. It was given to him by the philosopher and social scientist Friedrich Pollock, one of the founders of the *Institut für Sozialforschung* and the person to whom *Dialectic of Enlightenment* is dedicated.[41] Horkheimer and Leo Löwenthal, a sociologist closely associated with the *Frankfurter Schule*, were members of the *Schopenhauer Gesellschaft* when they were students.[42] In the 1960s, furthermore, Horkheimer wrote several essays in which he expressed the profound ways in which he was influenced by Schopenhauer [43] and even hung a picture of Schopenhauer in his room as director of the *Institut für Sozialforschung*.[44]

In these essays, Horkheimer praises several aspects of Schopenhauer's thinking, which I will briefly list here not only to provide a general overview of the reasons why the gap between Critical Theory and Schopenhauer is not as wide as is often suggested, but also to sketch the theoretical and historical context in which Schopenhauer and Adorno can be compared. Most of these aspects will therefore return in this book.

First, Horkheimer identifies with Schopenhauer's fight against 'superstition, intolerance and rational dogmatism' and places him in the tradition of critical enlightenment thinkers.[45] Second, he praises Schopenhauer's theory of perception. Not only does Horkheimer refer positively to Schopenhauer's idea that we do not perceive the world *as it is*, independently of our apparatus of perception, as an important argument against positivism, he also values the fact that Schopenhauer at the same time holds true to empiricist and materialist intuitions. Thereby, Schopenhauer both values and criticizes the tradition of German idealism and comes close to several of Marx's observations on the material dimension of the self, Horkheimer observes.[46] Third, Horkheimer praises Schopenhauer's deep suspicion of egotism.[47] Fourth, he values his influence on psychoanalysis, his understanding of the unconscious and especially his emphasis on the drive to self-preservation and the manner in which this drive manifests itself in the aforementioned egotistic tendencies.[48] Fifth, he argues that the radical negativity of Schopenhauer's approach to the world and humanity made it impossible to include him in the celebration of the state that characterized the ideology of National Socialism.[49] Sixth, Horkheimer claims that the horrors that were to come after Schopenhauer's lifetime show that he 'looked right into the heart of history'.[50] Seventh, Horkheimer identifies with Schopenhauer's emphasis on solidarity with suffering creatures and praises the negativity of his metaphysics; and eighth, values the fact that Schopenhauer positions this suffering in opposition to attempts at philosophical systematization – he specifically has Kant and Hegel in mind here.[51] Ninth, Horkheimer praises Schopenhauer's focus on the nature of existence and his concern with the possibility of finding happiness, again contrasting this emphasis on experience with the, in his view, more rationalistic and systematic theories of Kant and Hegel.[52] Tenth, Horkheimer discerns socialist and utopian traces in Schopenhauer's claim that the state is based on violence and that humanity will not have to be organized in nation-states once it overcomes its violent tendencies.[53] And lastly, Horkheimer deeply identifies with Schopenhauer's pessimism, defining his own guiding principle [*Grundsatz*] as follows: 'to be a theoretical pessimist and a practical optimist'.[54]

The Grand Hotel Abyss

Horkheimer's *Grundsatz* brings us to a third reason for comparing Schopenhauer and Adorno: Schopenhauer is not the only resident of the 'Grand Hotel Abyss'. Lukács states in his preface to *The Theory of the Novel*: 'a considerable part of the leading German intelligentsia, including Adorno, have taken up residence in the "Grand Hotel Abyss" which I described in connection with my critique of Schopenhauer.'[55] The egotism that Lukács accused Schopenhauer of echoes, in his reading, through Adorno's texts as well: instead of focusing on social antagonisms and ways to change the world for the better, the ego turns inwards in the writings of both and occupies itself only with musings on its own unhappiness, Lukács observes. Both Schopenhauer and Adorno, in other words, are accused of holding true to a crippling and passive form of pessimism.

One of the reasons for the fact that Lukács notices this similarity between Schopenhauer and Adorno's theories – and this is one of the main ideas that I will develop in this book – is that the powerlessness of the subject as approached from within the former's metaphysical system, being a mere slave to its metaphysical essence, returns in Adorno's theory in a historicized manner: Adorno's emphasis on the dominant nature of the social discourses he links to fascism, capitalism and what he defines as 'the culture industry' results in a diagnosis of the unfreedom of the modern self that in places equals Schopenhauer's metaphysical determinism.

Proust, Kafka, Beckett

Lukács' accusation of pessimistic egotism brings us to a fourth reason for comparing Schopenhauer and Adorno, which I want to discuss by looking at three authors who had a profound influence on Adorno's ideas and who were themselves influenced by Schopenhauer: the modernist writers Marcel Proust, Franz Kafka and Samuel Beckett. In 'Extorted reconciliation: On Georg Lukács' *Realism in Our Time*', Adorno discusses Lukács' reading of these authors – revolving around egotism again – and develops a powerful critique of Lukács' interpretation of art. I want to quote a lengthy passage from this essay, since Adorno here not only discusses one of the main methodological ideas behind his own philosophy, but also sheds light on the manner in which both his and Schopenhauer's works may be defended against the accusation of egotism:

> Proust decomposes the unity of the subject by means of the subject's introspection: the subject is ultimately transformed into an arena in which objective entities manifest themselves. Proust's individualistic work becomes the opposite of what Lukács criticizes it as being: it

> becomes anti-individualistic. The *monologue intérieur*, the worldlessness of modern art that Lukács is so indignant about, is both the truth and the illusion of a free-floating subjectivity. The truth, because in a world that is everywhere atomistic, alienation rules human beings and because – as we may concede to Lukács – they thereby become shadows. But the free-floating subject is an illusion, because the social totality is objectively prior to the individual; that totality becomes consolidated and reproduces itself in and through alienation, the social contradiction. The great avant-garde works of art cut through this illusion of subjectivity both by throwing the frailty of the individual into relief and by grasping the totality in the individual, who is a moment in the totality and yet can know nothing about it. In Joyce, Lukács thinks, Dublin, and in Kafka and Musil, the Hapsburg Monarchy, can be felt – *hors programme*, so to speak – as an atmospheric 'backcloth' to the Action……The concept of atmosphere is completely inappropriate for Kafka. It is derived from an impressionism that Kafka supersedes precisely through his objective tendency, which aims at historical essence. Even in Beckett – perhaps in Beckett most of all – where all concrete historical elements seem to have been eliminated and only primitive situations and modes of behavior are tolerated, the ahistorical facade is the provocative antithesis of the Being-as-such idolized by reactionary philosophy. The primitivism which is the abrupt point of departure for his works reveals itself to be the final phase of a regression… …The substantive content of a work of art can consist in the accurate and tacitly polemical representation of emerging meaninglessness, and that content can be lost when it is stated positively and hypostatized as existing, even if this occurs only indirectly… …Conceptions like Beckett's, however, are objectively polemical. Lukács falsifies them in describing them as the 'adoption of perversity and idiocy as types of the condition humaine' – following the practice of the film censor who blames the presentation for what it presents.… [Lukács blindness] derives from the fact that he stubbornly refuses to accord literary technique its rightful central place. Instead, he sticks indefatigably to what is narrated.[56]

Adorno observes, in other words, that Lukács overlooks the idea that describing a state of affairs in a radicalized and polemical manner *without* claiming that this state of affairs is wrong by explicitly linking it to specific historical conditions *nor* showing how and why this state of affairs can and should be changed, may result in a highly powerful and critical work of art. Even though Proust's *In Search of Lost Time* may appear as a celebration of individualism, for example, embodying a bourgeois existence permeated with ahistorical self-indulgence, Adorno argues that Proust's descriptions of the ego's fragmentation, of it 'becoming a shadow', a passive onlooker to an objective totality, shed light on the emptiness of this turn towards the ego's interior and thereby provide us with a critical analysis of this existence, intrinsically linked to the historical conditions under which this self-experience came into being.

I want to emphasize two aspects of the above-cited passage from Adorno's essay on Lukács. First, it provides us with a way to approach Adorno's reading of Schopenhauer. As briefly mentioned above, Adorno refers to Schopenhauer's ideas as embodying historical truths. This means that even though Schopenhauer's specific philosophical arguments may be flawed – as, for example, has been argued about his metaphysics – Adorno argues that his thought is valuable as a representation of the truth content of the times in which he lived. In *Minima Moralia*, for example, Adorno refers to Schopenhauer's claim that, in essence, the human self is unknowable since it is a manifestation of the ungraspable in-itself of the universe. Adorno historicizes this claim into the idea that it represents the subject's fragmented nature under bourgeois conditions, similar to his reading of Proust: 'the real self', he writes, 'has already become in the world what Schopenhauer recognized it to be in introspection, a phantom'.[57] Even though this may not be the case with all of Adorno's references to Schopenhauer, the mechanisms, tendencies and ideas that structure the latter's philosophy do present a historical way of thinking to which Adorno returns several times.

A second aspect that I want to emphasize concerns Adorno and Schopenhauer's pessimism. It is no coincidence that Lukács criticizes precisely Schopenhauer, Adorno, Proust, Kafka and Beckett. Schopenhauer had a profound influence on Beckett, who defined his philosophy as 'an intellectual justification of unhappiness – the greatest that has ever been attempted'.[58] He also influenced Kafka – especially his ideas on suffering, redemption and the religious notion of 'the indestructible'.[59] Proust read Schopenhauer as well and valued his ideas about the unconscious and the differences between voluntary and involuntary memory.[60]

Following Adorno's reading of Proust, Kafka and Beckett, I want to argue that Lukács misses the point that the methods both Schopenhauer and Adorno use and the manner in which they express their ideas contain critical value: their radical pessimism is aimed at providing a 'polemical representation' of the world that is radically critical in nature, precisely because it does not bow down to the demand to provide hope or to develop specific tools to change the world.

This point can be made more generally: a deeply pessimistic philosophy is not necessarily egotistic or uncritical in nature. In fact, I will argue in this book that both Schopenhauer and Adorno show us that it is precisely from a pessimistic point of view that the need to change the world or to seek happiness can be highlighted. They both transform a classic understanding of pessimism as an exclusive focus on despair into a dynamic and critical approach to the world, departing from Lukács' more one-dimensional definition of this doctrine.[61]

I want to return to Kafka to illustrate this idea. Adorno characterizes Kafka as follows:

> In the Middle Ages, Jews were tortured and executed 'perversely' – i.e. inversely.... Offenders were hung head down. Kafka, the land surveyor, photographs the earth's surface just as it must have appeared to these victims during the endless hours of their dying. It is for nothing less than such unmitigated torture that the perspective of redemption presents itself to him.[62]

Even though this 'photograph' Adorno describes is not accompanied by a sign saying 'this situation is wrong, but it can be changed in such and such a way', it is precisely the absence of such a sign that makes these 'photographs' critical and that urges us to think about methods to change the situations they depict.

We have to be very careful, however, not to approach art and philosophy as being similar in nature and to understand Schopenhauer and Adorno as just presenting us with a specific worldview, like Proust, Beckett and Kafka do. This would overlook the arguments they develop and the reasons that ground their ideas. The above-developed interpretation should therefore mainly be understood as a defence of the idea that the type of pessimism found in both Schopenhauer and Adorno's works does not necessarily follow from an egotistic point of view, but contains critical qualities that originate in its entwinement with the use of a specific style.

Corporeal suffering

This brings us to my fifth reason for comparing Schopenhauer and Adorno, which is thematic in nature: both share a concern with corporeality and, more specifically, with the suffering body. Together with a focus on the critical possibilities of their pessimism, this will form the main theme of this book. I will argue that important parts of the theories of both Schopenhauer and Adorno concern pain and, more specifically, extreme bodily suffering. This is the case, I aim to show, regarding several aspects of Schopenhauer's metaphysics, of Adorno's claims that the whole is the wrong and that the good cannot be known, and of their moral philosophies.

In line of Marx, who famously criticized Hegel's dialectics for 'standing on its head',[63] both Schopenhauer and Adorno focus on that which philosophy, in their view, tends to ignore: the materialistic dimensions of human existence and, more specifically, our bodies and their vulnerability to pain.

Characteristic for this discussion will be the following statement by Adorno, taken from his lectures on *Problems of Moral Philosophy*: 'We may not know what absolute good is or the absolute norm, we may not even know what man is or the human or humanity – but what the inhuman is we know very well indeed.'[64] For an important part, I will argue, negative statements like these refer to situations of extreme pain. These situations not only provide us with an absolute notion of the way things should *not* be, they also are so extreme that Adorno refuses to approach their normative value as in need of rationalization or justification. Indeed, I will argue, with reference to Jean Améry, Arne Johan Vetlesen and Elaine Scarry's observations on pain, that the corroding influence that extreme suffering has on the mind's ability to reflect plays an exemplary role in Adorno's ideas on the normative basis of moral philosophy.

Again, I believe, his above-cited characterization of Kafka as a land surveyor who 'photograph[s] the earth's surface just as it must have appeared to victims, hung head down, during the endless hours of their dying', is illustrative in this context: Adorno's philosophy, I will argue, and this is true of Schopenhauer's as well, is not written from a neutral perspective – if there is such a perspective at all – but from the radical perspective that comes with an emphasis on extreme bodily suffering and, like a corporeal response to pain, a 'concrete denunciation of the inhuman'. It is for this reason that Adorno keeps returning to what happened in Auschwitz when discussing practical philosophy and why he keeps referring, in the most normative passages of his writings, to the suffering of bodies.

This brings us to another similarity between Schopenhauer and Adorno's theories: their observations on the nature of aesthetic and metaphysical experiences. In the same passage on Kafka, Adorno describes how 'it is for nothing less than such unmitigated torture that the perspective of redemption presents itself to him'. Following this idea, I will argue that the phenomena of suffering and pain play an important role in 'methods of escape' from what Schopenhauer and Adorno both see as a prison-like world that diminishes the freedom of the self.[65] These methods of escape can be found in metaphysical and aesthetic experiences and play defining roles in their thinking, even though we will see that for Adorno, unlike for Schopenhauer, it is impossible to completely escape from a world that they both characterize as wrong.

Critical preliminaries

Before providing an overview of the structure of this book, it is important to notice that my discussion above may have given the impression that I want to overlook the many differences between Schopenhauer and Adorno. This is not the case: even though I indeed seek to discuss the similarities between these two authors, I also focus on the differences between their works. Not only is this necessary to do justice the specific nature of their theories, but I also believe that at those places where they do not agree with each other, interesting philosophical tensions arise that shed light on sometimes overlooked dimensions of their works.

The main observation that characterizes my analyses of these dimensions is that Schopenhauer arrives at conclusions that do not do justice to the complex nature of reality and the historically shaped experience of human beings, but that his arguments nevertheless provide us with insightful ideas that, in a more subtle and convincing form, return in Adorno's works.

It is furthermore important to stress that I do not want to argue that Schopenhauer and Adorno *exclusively* talk about pain. Nor do I want to reduce all of their ideas to this phenomenon or claim that my approach to their works is the most comprehensive. Regarding morality, for example, I will not argue that it is *only* pain that Adorno refers to as an 'absolute negative' or as 'the inhuman' in the passage quoted above. This would ignore the fact that he discusses many different social pathologies and covers several aspects of modern life in his works. My main interest is to highlight a specific dimension of both his and Schopenhauer's theories and to show that emphasizing this dimension may shed light on several famously problematic aspects of their works.

Another reason for not approaching both Schopenhauer and Adorno in a reductionist manner (by arguing that they only focus on pain and suffering) is that their writings do not really allow this. As we will see in this study, both authors do not provide us with theories of a completely closed and consistently systematic nature. Even though Schopenhauer develops a philosophical system that he himself understands as an organic whole,[66] I will argue that the different aspects of this system – embodied by the four books of *The World as Will and Representation* – contain too many contradictions and paradoxes to really approach his philosophy as unified and 'closed' or as revolving around one theme.

Adorno, furthermore, deliberately constructs a philosophy in which the attempt to systematically grasp the world and its phenomena is replaced by a focus on philosophy as a critical and often fragmented endeavour. Instead of mirroring the false ideology he criticizes, which pulls everything different, everything 'other' into itself, Adorno seeks to construct a philosophy that consists of 'fragments', 'constellations' or 'prisms'. This does not mean that his philosophy is not systematic *at all* or that it is completely fragmentary, but it does mean that there is an *openness* about his thought that allows me, as I aim to show, to emphasize a specific dimension of his ideas without reducing them to this same dimension.[67]

The fact that I highlight one dimension of Schopenhauer and Adorno's ideas also means that I will overlook other aspects of their thought or will not emphasize the importance of these aspects enough. Even though I try to be as inclusive as possible – mentioning which aspects I may overlook, which interpretations my focus on the phenomena of pain and suffering may contradict, or which passages and claims by Schopenhauer and Adorno themselves may undermine my own interpretation – it is already at this point that I want to acknowledge that my specific approach to their ideas limits my perspective.

This emphasis on one specific theme – pain, suffering and our ways of dealing with them – furthermore means that I may not pay enough attention to the way both Schopenhauer and Adorno's ideas have changed over time. Even though the theories of both remain fairly consistent throughout their works, these works are, of course, characterized by subtle shifts in focus, inspired by new ideas, experiences or insights. This is the case, for example, regarding Schopenhauer's references to the body: even though his earlier texts contain many naturalistic tendencies, in his later writings he reduces mental capacities more and more to bodily functions.[68] In the case of Adorno, I believe that we mainly find such a difference in approach between his books and essays on the one hand and his published lectures on the other. In these lectures Adorno tends to be much clearer than in his other writings, providing many examples that often clarify the denser and obscurer nature of his books and essays. In this study, I will therefore frequently refer to these lectures.

Another problematic aspect of this book is that I may be too uncritical of both Schopenhauer and Adorno from a general point of view. I therefore try to shed a critical light on their ideas by confronting them with each other as well as discussing them in light of theories of other thinkers, like Immanuel Kant and Christine Korsgaard. Nevertheless, it remains true that I mainly compare the two and therefore focus only on their works.

As a last preliminary point, it is important to mention that I do not seek to answer the questions described above in light of Kafka's story in a definitive manner. Not only are these questions far too complex to be answered within the scope of this book – if they can be answered at all – but I also believe, mainly following Adorno, that raising and discussing these questions is valuable in itself since it already forces us to reflect on ourselves and the conditions we find ourselves in. Instead of arriving at clear and definitive answers or explanations, it is precisely this reflection that I understand as one of the most important ethical demands we have to set ourselves: not to be content with the situations in which we live but to keep questioning and re-evaluating our world; educating ourselves and those around us by relying on a worldview that forces us to be critical of others and, even more importantly, ourselves and our own tendencies, ideas and actions. And as I argue in this study, this demand remains relevant as long as there is unnecessary suffering.

Structure

This book consists of two parts and nine chapters. In Part I, containing five chapters, I discuss the arguments that result in both Schopenhauer and Adorno's claims that the world, as a whole, is wrong. In Part II, containing four chapters, I develop interpretations of their ideas on morality, happiness and salvation. These interpretations follow from the analyses developed in Part I.

Part I can be read as an overview of and an introduction to the philosophies of Schopenhauer and Adorno, also by those who are not familiar with their works. Part II contains more detailed and in-depth discussions of their specific ideas.

The first three chapters of Part I revolve around Schopenhauer. I discuss his ideas on the world-as-representation, which I do by briefly referring to Merleau-Ponty's and Adorno's observations on perception (Chapter 2); then I analyse his not-unproblematic understanding of the metaphysical world-as-will (Chapter 3); I conclude with an analysis of Schopenhauer's pessimism (Chapter 4). In this latter chapter I mainly focus on the relation between rationality and corporeality, since Schopenhauer's pessimism is rooted in the tension between these two poles of human existence, I argue.

In Chapter 5 I discuss how Adorno transforms Schopenhauer's metaphysical observations on the world into an equally bleak historical diagnosis of modernity. This discussion is followed by an analysis of Adorno's ideas on the tension between rationality and embodiment (Chapter 6).

Part II begins with analyses of Schopenhauer's moral philosophy, which I contrast with Korsgaard's ideas on rational endorsement (Chapter 7). In Chapter 8 I discuss Adorno's thoughts on morality. In these chapters, a concern with bodily suffering and with the phenomenon of compassion plays a central role and is discussed in light of Kant's practical philosophy. In order to shed light on Adorno's observations on suffering, I also refer to Elaine Scarry, Jean Améry and Arne Johan Vetlesen's observations on pain.

The last two chapters revolve around 'methods of escape' from a world that both Schopenhauer and Adorno characterize as wrong. For the former, these are found in a state of salvation that borders on mysticism (Chapter 9); the latter places them in glimpses of happiness found in childhood memories, brief experiences of peace, and a rather vague understanding of a better society (Chapter 10). Both, I also show, argue that art and especially music play an essential role in providing us with references to a state of being that is different and that consists mainly of a changed relationship between subject and object.

Almost every chapter of this book begins with a short analysis of an artist or an artwork, as this does with the discussion of Franz Kafka's *In the Penal Colony*. I do this because several of the themes and experiences I refer to are particular and embedded in complex dimensions of human life. I therefore find discussing the less systematic and, to borrow a term from Adorno, 'micrological'[69] field of the arts helpful in illustrating these topics. I also do this because it ties in with the methodologies of Schopenhauer and Adorno themselves. Both authors frequently refer to writers, playwrights, poets, composers and painters to highlight observations or illustrate and strengthen arguments.

Part I

Determinism, Rationality, Embodiment

2
A Paradox of Transcendence and Immanence

Introduction

In *Schopenhauer on the Character of the World: The Metaphysics of Will*, John E. Atwell characterizes Arthur Schopenhauer as follows:

> It would not be an exaggeration to dub Schopenhauer *the* philosopher of the body. To a greater extent than anyone before his time ... he makes the body – that is, one's own body (*der eigene Leib*) – the primary focus and indispensable condition of all philosophical inquiry. If required to give a single answer to the philosophizing subject's question, 'What am I' Schopenhauer would surely reply, 'I am body,' though, he would just as surely add, 'in more than one way.' He therefore deposes the mind from the throne of philosophical investigation and installs in its place – the place the mind has occupied since at least the time of Descartes – the body, which plays the crucial role in theory of knowledge ..., in ethics ... and in metaphysics proper.[1]

In this chapter, I will follow Atwell's observations by developing an introductory analysis of Schopenhauer's theory of perception and the role that the body plays in it.

This aspect of his philosophy, which he develops in the first book of *The World as Will and Representation*, does not directly play a role in his analyses of the phenomena of pain and suffering, the main themes of this study. However, it is crucial to first focus on Schopenhauer's epistemology for four reasons. First, in order to discuss his understanding of the world-as-will, on which his ideas on suffering, the unconscious, compassion and the powerlessness of rationality rest, we need to shed light on his analysis of the world we perceive, which he calls the 'world-as-representation' and which he approaches as 'the other', as a *negative image* of the world-as-will. Any analysis of Schopenhauer's philosophy, in other words, needs to start with a discussion of the 'world-as-representation'. Second, discussing Schopenhauer's observations on the role that the body plays in perception is necessary to arrive at an understanding of the important role that corporeality and bodily suffering play in his philosophy as a whole. Third, his claim that our epistemological apparatus necessarily makes us perceive the world as permeated with the *principium individuationis* and therefore as consisting of separate objects, plays a crucial role in his moral philosophy and returns as well in Adorno's moral observations. Fourth, Schopenhauer's conclusion that perception is irrational in nature returns in Chapter 4 in my analysis of his ideas about rationality.

I will discuss Schopenhauer's epistemology in this chapter by focusing on a fundamental contradiction within his discussion of the world-as-representation. I will show that this contradiction greatly compromises the idealist framework within which his understanding of this world is initially constructed and forces us to conclude that he defends a kind of idealism that has strong naturalistic tendencies.

Without trying to deemphasize the problematic nature of Schopenhauer's theory of perception, I will end this chapter with a brief discussion of Adorno and Merleau-Ponty's observations on epistemology and argue that the contradictions inherent to Schopenhauer's theory of perception highlight a problematic aspect of the field of epistemology *itself*, revolving around the role that the body plays in perception.

The world-as-representation

Schopenhauer opens his chief work with the following claim: 'The world is my representation: this is a truth valid with reference to every living and knowing being.'[2] He bases this claim on an analysis he developed in *The Fourfold Root of the Principle of Sufficient Reason* (*Über die vierfache Wurzel des Satzes vom zureichenden Grunde*), his doctoral dissertation of 1813, presented at the University of Jena and published in a revised form in 1847.[3] Below, I will provide a brief summary of the main ideas behind this work. This summary will be quite technical and dry, but is necessary in order to understand the manner in which Schopenhauer tries to 'smuggle' the body into an epistemology that he formulates within a framework defined by the tradition of German idealism.

The Fourfold Root of the Principle of Sufficient Reason revolves around the 'principle of sufficient reason', which Schopenhauer defines as follows: 'the Principle of Sufficient Reason is the *principle of all explanation: to explain a thing* means, to reduce its given existence to some form or other of the Principle of Sufficient Reason, in accordance with which form that existence or connection necessarily is that which it is.'[4] As the title suggests, this principle has four 'roots', each referring to a different class of objects; first, empirical, intuitive representations; second, abstract, non-empirical concepts; third, *a priori* pure intuitions like geometrical objects; and fourth, the subject in volition known in self-consciousness.

Within the scope of the current chapter and its focus on embodiment, only a discussion of the first class is relevant, since it is this class that forms the most explicit 'other' of the 'world-as-will'. This first class consists of everyday and *individual* objects like stones or tables, which Schopenhauer distinguishes from conceptuality and from abstract thought in general, as we will see.

As mentioned above, Schopenhauer's epistemology is formulated within the tradition of German idealism, which means that he defends the idea that the perceived world is dependent on a perceiving subject that provides this world with its form and structure. He argues that objects have two *formal properties* – temporality and spatiality – that are imposed upon them by the inner sense (time) and outer sense (space) of the perceiving subject.[5] He refers to these properties as well as 'a priori fundamental intuitions'[6] and bases this claim mainly on a phenomenological analysis of that which makes an object into an object as it *appears* to the subject.

What defines an object as a *real object* (like a stone or a table) according to his analysis, is its *permanence* or *durability* as an individual thing. It does not suddenly disappear or come into existence 'out of nowhere'. Time, Schopenhauer observes, therefore forms a necessary property of real objects. However, he argues, this permanence – its staying the same during a period of time – can 'only be recognized by contrast with the changes going on in other objects coexistent with it'.[7] And this 'coexistence', in turn, can only be perceived once Space is added as a necessary formal property because 'in mere Time, all things *follow one another,* and in mere Space all things are *side by side*'.[8] Hence, he claims, empirical representations – real objects – 'grow out of' the 'intimate union' of Space and Time.[9]

However, these two formal properties, Schopenhauer then argues, are *in themselves* not enough to constitute the world we perceive: we would then only 'have' the *empty* forms of Time and Space. These forms, in other words, need to be 'filled with something', as F.C. White terms this process in an insightful article on Schopenhauer's first book,[10] which happens when what Schopenhauer calls the *faculty of the Understanding* imposes the category of *causality* on the world. The faculty of the Understanding interprets the data it 'receives' in some way or another as *caused* by objects in the empirical world and reconstructs these data, as it were, 'into' the material and particular objects it perceives.

In a peculiar move, Schopenhauer identifies the category of causality with 'matter' *itself*. This claim is based on the argument that an object is only material once it can *cause* changes, once it can *causally influence* other objects, and once it is *understood* as affecting our senses *causally*: only by reconstructing the data that the subject receives as *caused* by a specific object in front of it, he argues, does the material world come about. This means that Schopenhauer not only understands causal efficacy as a *criterion* of materiality, he identifies the *content* of sense experience – *matter* – with 'causality' as well, making both its form and its content subjective in nature.

The law of causality, Schopenhauer then concludes, is the *necessary underlying principle* of the interconnectedness of objects in the world, forming the first 'root' of the principle of sufficient reason, which he calls the *Principle of Sufficient Reason of Becoming*.[11]

The 'intuitive' and 'quite direct process'[12] by which the perception of an object comes about, according to Schopenhauer, can thus be summarized as follows: in some way or another, the intellect 'receives' time-less, space-less and causally inactive data in forms such as colours and smells – these data, which he sometimes refers to as 'raw materials',[13] are *subjective* in nature because they are particular sensations 'in' the subject – and imposes the *subjective* forms of space and time as well as the *subjective* category of causality on them, thereby constituting the particular object perceived in front of the subject. This means that empirical reality is, by definition, characterized by the *principium individuationis*:[14] it consists of individual and separate objects. And these objects, Schopenhauer concludes in an idealistic fashion, are *subjective* in nature; perception is 'intellectual in character',[15] and empirical reality is 'ideal'.[16]

Idealism and naturalism

Kant

This briefly described chain of arguments has several problematic aspects.[17] One of these is captured by the following question: what is the specific *content* of our sense experience and how does the subject receive it? On the one hand, we have seen that Schopenhauer refers to a 'raw material' that is 'given to the intellect' by the senses and that provides it with *matter* that the intellect, in turn, shapes into the world it perceives. These references to 'raw material' imply that there is 'something' external to the world-as-representation on which our perception is based. Schopenhauer therefore claims that he does not defend scepticism about the existence of the world-as-representation and argues that even though what he calls 'theoretical egoism' cannot be refuted by proofs, it is nevertheless an absurd position.[18] The world we perceive *is there*, he states, and its denial is a 'sceptical sophism' that should not be taken seriously.[19]

Paradoxically, however, we have also seen that Schopenhauer equates the subjective category of causality with matter *itself*. This implies that the 'raw material' that is 'given' to the senses is subjective in nature, which means in turn that there might be no 'ground' for the world-as-representation independent of the subject that perceives this world: everything we perceive might be an illusion. By equating causality with matter, in other words, Schopenhauer makes the distinction between a perception and the world of objects disappear, and suggests that the world-as-representation is *completely* subjective in nature.[20] In several passages, he indeed suggests that the world we perceive is, ultimately, an illusion, and refers positively to the works of Berkeley and to Eastern scriptures according to which 'existence and perceptibility are convertible terms'.[21]

I want to argue that it is the vagueness surrounding this issue that eventually waters down the idealist nature of some of Schopenhauer's observations (revolving around the idea that the world we perceive is completely dependent on the subject), which provides him with the possibility of introducing the body into his epistemology. But before I discuss the specific way in which this happens, I first want to provide a brief overview of Schopenhauer's reading of Kant's epistemology. Even though the scope of this chapter does not allow me to discuss the intricacies of Kant's philosophy of perception in detail (I am mainly concerned with Schopenhauer's ideas on the body and the role it plays in his epistemology), I believe that looking at Schopenhauer's understanding of Kant provides us with several important observations regarding the former's analysis of idealism.

Kant famously tried to solve Hume's sceptical question of whether 'the concept of causality could be thought by reason *a priori*, and consequently, whether it possessed an inner truth'[22] by arguing that 'causality' is a pure concept of the understanding that makes experience of an objective world possible.[23] Kant herewith aimed to remove sceptical arguments about the existence of the perceived world by reasoning *a priori* and by transcendentally constructing the conditions of the possibility of this world.

Schopenhauer departs from Kant's epistemology by developing observations of a phenomenological and not of a transcendental nature: he does not analyse the conditions that make the existence of the world-as-representation possible, but merely looks at the way in which this world *appears* to the subject. In an appendix to the first volume of his chief work, Schopenhauer indeed criticizes Kant's philosophy for lacking a 'grand, classical simplicity' and Kant himself for having a 'peculiar liking for symmetry'.[24] Instead of *directly* analysing the way we perceive the world, Schopenhauer observes, Kant took a 'reflective detour' by focusing on the rational and conceptual nature of the perceiving subject, constructing the table of judgements and 'violently' forcing 'all things in the world and everything that occurs in man in the symmetry of that table'.[25] Schopenhauer therefore dismisses Kant's arguments, does away with all categories but causality, and concludes that the process by which the world-as-representation comes about is 'irrational' in nature and devoid of conceptuality: 'the understanding is in itself irrational, even in man. Reason can always only *know*; perception remains free from its influence, and belongs to the understanding alone.'[26]

I want to illustrate Schopenhauer's phenomenological approach to perception by focusing on his analysis of causality. His main defence of the idea that this category structures our perception of the world consists of the observation that it cannot be 'thought away' *from a phenomenological point of view*: causality *has to* be imposed by the Understanding, he argues, since without it the data that the subject 'receives' could not be reconstructed into a material object existing in front of this same subject. Furthermore, if we did not 'have' the category of causality, we would only perceive unconnected states of spatial appearances that succeed each other in time, he observes. Causality, Schopenhauer's main argument therefore goes, has to be *added* in order to understand these states as being *caused* by other states and in order to produce the causally structured world we *already* perceive. Schopenhauer hereby merely affirms Hume's scepticism and argues that the subject, in some way or another, has to 'add' the category of causality to the world because otherwise we would not be able to make sense of the way in which we happen to perceive this world. According to Schopenhauer, in other words, causality is 'just' a mental category and therefore relative to the subject, whereas in Kant's view the subject forms the transcendental condition of the existence of the perceived world.

In light of these observations, it has been suggested that Schopenhauer's epistemology does not revolve around questions regarding the *existence* of the world-as-representation, but around the idea that this world is *relative* to the experiencing subject.[27] According to this interpretation, which I find convincing, Schopenhauer's phenomenological approach to perception is aimed at the specific way in which the subject relates to the world in which it lives and which it perceives, and stays away from transcendental forms of reasoning or claims regarding the existence of this world. This interpretation implies, however, that we have to overlook those passages in which Schopenhauer claims that the world-as-representation is a complete illusion.

Paradoxes

This brings us to the most problematic aspect of Schopenhauer's case for idealism: the fact that he does not seek to develop *a priori* arguments that transcendentally guarantee the existence of the world as it appears to the subject but merely analyses the way in which this subject experiences a world in which it already lives and which it already perceives, makes it possible for him to infuse and at places even *base* his analysis of perception on *naturalistic observations* of an *a posteriori* nature. He frequently refers to the 'perceiving subject' as the *brain* of embodied creatures, arguing that the brain 'interprets' the sense data it 'receives' from the body's five senses, and defining perception as 'a function of the brain, which the brain no more learns by experience than the stomach to digest, or the liver to secrete bile'.[28] One of the examples he often refers to in order to substantiate his claim that perception is subjective consists of the observation that we have two eyes but only one visual field, concluding that the Understanding 'steps in' by imposing the law of causality, thereby 'reconstructing' the one object that is eventually perceived as the 'cause' of the two streams of data that the brain receives from the eyes.[29] Schopenhauer also frequently refers to optical illusions – like the moon appearing to be bigger on the horizon – as an argument for the claim that there is a difference between the world we *perceive* and the world *as it is*.[30]

This introduction of naturalistic observations renders the basis of Schopenhauer's idealism highly problematic and forms another argument for the idea that he mainly develops a rather pragmatic and phenomenological analysis of the way in which the subject, *as an embodied being*, experiences the world in which it lives. Instead of understanding the world of objects, including the body and the brain, as completely dependent on and structured by the subject, Schopenhauer pulls this latter subject into the natural world and reduces it to the status of an empirical entity: 'man is concerned merely with his own representations, which as such are the work of his brain; therefore their conformity to law is merely the mode or manner in which the function of his brain alone can be carried out, in other words, the form of his representing.'[31]

Another illustration of this 'naturalization' of the subject appears in Schopenhauer's analysis of the *development* of the ability to perceive a world-as-representation within the context of a theory that, in certain respects, comes close to Darwin's ideas on evolution:[32]

> The higher we ascend in the scale of animals, the greater number and perfection of the senses we find, till at last we have all five; these are found in a small number of invertebrate animals, but they only become universal in the vertebrate. The brain and its function, the understanding, develop proportionately, and the object now gradually presents itself more and more distinctly and completely and even already in connection with other objects.[33]

Above, we have seen that Schopenhauer claims that the Understanding is irrational in nature. Now, he also dismisses the idea that human beings perceive a structured and 'objective' world, not dependent on instincts or desires, and replaces this idea with the claim that *both* human and non-human animals perceive the *same* world because both are embodied creatures with bodily senses and a nervous system. Furthermore, he herewith leaves open the possibility that animals with different sense organs (like the electrical sensory system of sharks or the echolocation used by bats) experience this same world of objects in different ways.

This naturalization of the idea that the subject forms the condition of the perceived world results in paradoxical arguments like the following: 'the existence of this whole world remains for ever dependent on that first eye that opened, were it even that of an insect. For such an eye necessarily brings about knowledge, for which and in which alone the whole world is, and without which it is not even conceivable.'[34] Of course, this 'opening eye' *already* has to be in the world *as a material object* in order to perceive this world and cannot *at the same* time be the *condition* of its own existence *as matter*. A similar paradox, which Spierling defines in his introduction to Schopenhauer's lectures on the *Metaphysik der Sitten* as 'die Welt ist im Kopf, und der Kopf ist in der Welt',[35] is found in the statements that follow the above cited first sentence of *The World as Representation*. Schopenhauer there writes that the subject 'does not know a sun and an earth, but only an eye that sees a sun, a hand that feels an earth'.[36]

Biological idealism

An important motive underlying Schopenhauer's case for idealism is desire to do justice to the natural sciences and to the realm of the corporeal. At places, he seems to be aware of the paradox that is inherent to his epistemology and claims: 'the possibility of knowing the world of perception is to be found in two conditions',[37] the first being the experiencing subject ('the world of perception exists only for it and through it'[38]), the second being 'the sensibility of animal bodies'.[39] However, he does not seem to find this paradox overly problematic and defines it as an 'antinomy of our faculty of knowledge' that 'simply' cannot be solved: 'we see, on the one hand, the existence of the whole world necessarily dependent on the first knowing being, however imperfect it be; on the other hand, this first knowing animal just as necessarily wholly dependent on a long chain of causes and effects which has preceded it, and in which it itself appears as a small link.'[40]

In an excellent discussion of the tension between idealism and naturalism in Schopenhauer's philosophy, Julian Young insightfully argues that this paradox is partly caused by the fact that in the times in which Schopenhauer lived idealism was 'uncontroversial'.[41] He concludes that Schopenhauer develops a 'bio-physiological version of Kantianism' that can be defined as 'biological idealism'.[42] Schopenhauer, in other words, accepted the doctrine of idealism – as most philosophers did in his time – but *also* tried to do justice to medical and biological observations on the human being as a body, as a natural object not fundamentally different from non-human animals.[43]

Combined with the phenomenological and empirical nature of his arguments, this resulted in a notion of the world-as-representation that does not transcendentally guarantee the existence of the external world, but that is a product of a material brain that is embedded in an already existing material world and that merely structures this world in a certain way. His idealism hereby rests on arguments of a naturalistic nature, and follows, for example, from the observations that the brain structures the data it receives from two eyes into one visual field and that animals with different sense organs experience the world of objects differently from human beings.

The truth moment of Schopenhauer's epistemology

Christopher Janaway insightfully claims that Schopenhauer defends a position we can define as 'correlativism'[44] and argues that even though Schopenhauer is unsuccessful in reconciling 'subjective' points of view (regarding the way the world appears to the subject) with 'objective' observations (regarding the nature of the sense organs and the brain) he is not alone in this failure, which reflects an irreconcilable difference between the experience we have of the world as subjects on the one hand, and our existence as objects in a natural world of objects on the other.[45] The paradox underlying Schopenhauer's discussion of the notion of a world-as-representation, in other words, reflects a *truth moment* about epistemology as a philosophical doctrine.

In the following, I want to embed Janaway's important observation in a brief discussion of the arguments developed in two works: Theodor W. Adorno's *Against Epistemology. A Metacritique: Studies in Husserl and the Phenomenological Antinomies* (*Zur Metakritik der Erkenntnistheorie*), which he began writing during his studies in England, left unfinished and eventually published in 1956, and Maurice Merleau-Ponty's 1945 magnum opus *Phenomenology of Perception* (*Phénoménologie de la perception*).

Adorno

Schopenhauer's refusal to solve the paradox underlying his epistemology by claiming that it forms an irresolvable 'antinomy of our faculty of knowledge'[46] touches on a problem that Adorno describes as inherent to epistemology as well. Adorno bases this argument on the observation that the notion of a transcendental subject is not able to do justice to naturalistic observations on the role of the material body in cognition:

> The anathema against 'naturalism' does not save epistemology from having recourse...to the apparatus of sense-perception, the sense-organs. According to the ground rules of epistemology, however, such organs are a bit of the thing world. And thus epistemology gets caught in the *ὕστερον πρότερον*. The insistent demand to exclude the sense organs, as well as the individual person who bears them, from constitutional analysis, is just a bit of apologetic strategy....Seeing could not be conceived without eyes nor hearing without ears. The *μετάβασις είς ἄλλο γένος*, of deriving the given, the primary matter of cognition, as a consequence of the sense organs, viz. of what they themselves are meant to constitute, is no corrigible error of thought. Its unavoidability leads the starting point of philosophy of immanence to its own falsehood.[47]

Adorno tries to show how corporeity forms a kind of 'other' to the classical notion of the transcendental subject; an 'other' that cannot be neglected. If we take sensibility seriously, he argues, the transcendental subject 'cannot be isolated from the sense organs at all'.[48] Since the subject, understood within what Adorno calls 'philosophies of immanence' – in Schopenhauer's case, the idea of a world-as-representation *completely* dependent on the subject – is 'cut off' from the world it perceives, which, paradoxically, *includes* the body and its sense organs, it remains an abstraction, an entity floating in thin air: 'nothing can be given to a "pure" transcendental subject. For that subject is a determination of thought, a product of abstraction.... The transcendental subject itself is supposed to be cut off from the given by the ontological difference which should disappear in the construction of the subject.'[49] Adorno therefore concludes that 'the body should be of immeasurable significance for the starting point of phenomenology'.[50]

Adorno hereby affirms Schopenhauer's above-cited observation that the understanding has to 'start with something',[51] with what Schopenhauer calls the 'sensitivity of animal bodies': there has to be some kind of *friction* with a world 'surrounding' the perceiver in order to make sense of the idea of perception at all. In the second volume of *The World as Will and Representation*, Schopenhauer indeed discusses materialism as a necessary half of the construction of a theory of the subject: 'materialism also has its justification. It is just as true that the knower is a product of matter as that matter is a mere representation of the knower; but it is also just as one-sided. For materialism is the philosophy of the subject who forgets to take account of himself.'[52]

The second half of this statement, concerning the ideas that there has to be, to put it Kantian, some sort of 'unity of apperception' and that the subject influences and structures the way it perceives the world, is affirmed by Adorno in his essay 'On Subject and Object'.[53] He there criticizes the physiological and empiricist side of this debate for following from a 'slavish confidence in the external world existing precisely as it appears this side of critique, an anthropological state devoid of the self-consciousness that first crystallizes in the context of the relationship leading from knowledge back to the knower'.[54]

I return to Adorno's ideas on epistemology in Chapters 5 and 6. These ideas entail more than hitherto discussed and are embedded in Adorno's understanding of negative dialectics, art and metaphysical experience. Furthermore, Adorno argues that the perceiving subject is permeated with historical and social categories and that the way we perceive and experience the world is influenced by the culture and society in which we live; his epistemology is infused with Hegelian observations that Schopenhauer's ahistorical ideas lack. Nevertheless, in his and Horkheimer's *Dialectic of Enlightenment* the 'circularity' of Schopenhauer's view on perception is praised as illustrating the 'intermeshed relationship of subject and object' that the 'official logical consistency' of neo-Kantian schools misses.[55]

Merleau-Ponty

In Merleau-Ponty's *Phenomenology of Perception* we find a critique of traditional theories of perception that originates in the same observations Adorno makes in *Against Epistemology*, based on the insight that Kant's focus on the constitutive role of consciousness 'caused him to overlook the phenomenon of the body and that of the thing'.[56] He observes in a passage in which he refers to Marx's famous line about Hegel, mentioned in Chapter 1:

> It is true, as Marx says, that history does not walk on its head, but it is also true that it does not think with its feet. Or one should say that it is neither its 'head' nor its 'feet' that we have to worry about, but its body.[57]

Unlike Adorno, who is wary of bridging the gap between mind and body for reasons I discuss in Chapters 5 and 6, Merleau-Ponty tries to do justice to the two 'moments' of Schopenhauer's philosophy – bodily sensation and experiencing self – by seeking a (not unproblematic) middle ground between the two, developing a phenomenology that revolves around the idea that body and consciousness are fundamentally entwined *within* our 'lived experience' of the world and ourselves.[58] Like Adorno, Merleau-Ponty therewith argues that the ideas both of pure empiricism and of pure idealism are abstractions that negate the truth moment of their 'other': neither can be postulated as a 'first'.[59]

In his essay 'The Primacy of Perception', an elaboration of the underlying ideas and thoughts of *Phenomenology of Perception*, Merleau-Ponty argues that this approach forces him to embrace a paradox:

> The perceived thing itself is paradoxical; it exists only in so far as someone can perceive it. I cannot even for an instant imagine an object in itself. As Berkeley said, if I attempt to imagine some place in the world which has never been seen, the very fact that I imagine it makes me present at that place. I thus cannot conceive a perceptible place in which I am not myself present.[60]

We can put this paradox in Schopenhauer's terms: the world is dependent on the first eye that opens, but is on the other hand also *already* there when this eye opens – the eye itself is, after all, *already* part of a world that presents itself again *to* this eye. Merleau-Ponty insightfully concludes: 'there is a paradox of immanence and transcendence in perception. Immanence, because the perceived object cannot be foreign to him who perceives; transcendence, because it always contains something more than what is actually given.'[61]

Conclusion

In this chapter, I have looked at Atwell's claim that Schopenhauer is *the* philosopher of the body by discussing what Schopenhauer calls the 'world-as-representation' and focusing on several of the contradictions and paradoxes it contains. Whereas his theory of perception originates within an idealist framework, it remains unclear what precisely the nature is of the world that we perceive and what the content is of our experience. Instead of transcendentally guaranteeing the existence of the world, Schopenhauer develops arguments of a phenomenological, pragmatic and empirical nature that result in a system that Young defines as 'biological idealism'.

Without trying to deemphasize the problematic nature of his theory of perception, I want to conclude that Merleau-Ponty's 'paradox of immanence and transcendence' illustrates the idea that the paradox underlying Schopenhauer's world-as-representation enlightens a fundamental problem of epistemology *itself*, which mainly arises if one seeks to take the role of the body seriously. As we have seen, this aspect of Schopenhauer's epistemology was praised by Adorno, who writes in *Against Epistemology*: 'no sheer sensation can be detached from perception in the real life of consciousness. The two can be distinguished only by dint of a theory which posits sensation as a placeholder for the thing-in-itself.'[62]

Schopenhauer's peculiar mixture of idealism and naturalism, in other words, teaches us that we have to take two claims into account: that we encounter a world as a sentient body *and* that we grasp this world as structured by the experiencing self, which means that this world is always already subjective in nature. It teaches us that the idea of a bodiless subject is a philosophical and abstract invention and that, by detaching the senses from the body, we push the corporeal into the realm of the unknown.

3
The World-as-Will

Introduction

The paintings of the Anglo-Irish artist Francis Bacon often depict raw meat, bodies torn apart by inner demons, conflicting desires and unseen forces that distort their faces and limbs. One of his most famous paintings is *Three Studies for Figures at the Base of a Crucifixion* (1944). This painting forms a meditation on the image of the suffering body of Christ as, on the one hand, the symbol of a religion revolving around the idea that suffering is inherent in the human condition and, on the other hand, as a depiction of the sometimes evil nature of men, symbolized by a torture device designed to bring suffering and death to the body and make its pain into a spectacle. The painting embodies Schopenhauer's observations that 'in the New Testament, the world is presented as a vale of tears, life as a process of purification, and the symbol of Christianity is an instrument of torture'[1] and that 'in its innermost core, Christianity bears the truth that suffering (the Cross) is the real purpose of life'.[2]

In his famous study of Bacon, Wieland Schmied describes the painter's fascination with the crucifix as revolving around 'the motif of meat, the raw, bleeding flesh of the slaughterhouse and the butcher's slab, a sight that affected Bacon like almost no other and that was to become his personal metaphor of death'.[3] In Gilles Deleuze's study of Bacon, furthermore, we find the following interesting passage:

> Meat is not dead flesh; it retains all the sufferings and assumes all the colors of living flesh. It manifests such convulsive pain and vulnerability, but also such delightful invention, color, and acrobatics. Bacon does not say, 'Pity the beasts,' but rather that every man who suffers

> is a piece of meat. Meat is the common zone of man and beast, their zone of indiscernibility; it is a 'fact,' a state where the painter identifies with the objects of his horror and of his compassion.[4]

Deleuze illustrates this powerful observation with a quote taken from an interview with the artist himself: 'I've always been very moved by pictures about slaughterhouses and meat, and to me they belong very much to the whole thing of the Crucifixion ... Of course, we are meat, we are potential carcasses. If I go into a butcher shop, I always think it's surprising that I wasn't there instead of the animal.'[5] Indeed, Bacon painted the carcasses of animals nailed to a wall like Christ was nailed to the cross, blurring the line between humans and animals by focusing on the tissue that makes us equal to animals: flesh and its ability to suffer.

In the following, I will focus on these themes as they return in Schopenhauer's metaphysics. In Chapter 2 we have seen that Schopenhauer's epistemology contains several problematic contradictions, one of the most important following from his attempt to include the body into what he calls the 'world-as-representation'. In this chapter I will show that his metaphysical system, revolving around the 'world-as-will', contains several highly problematic aspects as well. Again, most of these follow from his concern with corporeity. This time, however, it is not the body as it forms part of our epistemological apparatus that poses a problem; instead, Schopenhauer now focuses on the body as a striving, feeling and suffering entity.

Whereas I have argued in Chapter 2 that his epistemology does show us something about the role that the body can and should play in our ideas about perception, I will argue in this chapter that Schopenhauer's metaphysics, although flawed, does contain an interesting side as well, revolving around intercorporeity and compassion.

A key to the world

Two worlds

To a certain extent, Schopenhauer's analysis of the world-as-representation, discussed in Chapter 2, forms a mere prelude to a development of his notion of the world-as-will: with the introduction of this latter world he expresses an overarching interest in a distinction between two 'worlds' that, in its generality, overshadows the intrinsic and detailed problems of his discussion of the world-as-representation.[6] Georg Simmel insightfully points this out, in contrast with Kant, in his famous study of Schopenhauer and Nietzsche:

> Kant senses reality as a category which produces experience, whereas Schopenhauer, who thirsts for the metaphysical absolute, senses reality in opposition to experience. For Kant, the phenomenality of experience is the point of arrival.... For Schopenhauer, phenomenality becomes a mere tool that inscribes a locus for the absoluteness of an ulterior experience.[7]

The general nature of this distinction between two worlds becomes apparent at those places where Schopenhauer links it to a wide range of authors that have each developed rather different understandings of this dualism. In the first sentence of *The Fourfold Root of the Principle of Sufficient Reason*, for example, he argues that this idea has been developed by both 'the divine Plato and the marvellous Kant',[8] observing in *The World as Will and Representation*: 'Kant's greatest merit is the distinction of the phenomenon from the thing-in-itself, based on the proof that between things and us there always stands the intellect, and that on this account they cannot be known according to what they may be in themselves.'[9] Schopenhauer writes:

> [Kant] propounded, quite originally and in an entirely new way, the same truth, found from a new aspect and a new path, which Plato untiringly repeats, and generally expresses in his language as follows. This world that appears to the senses has no true being, but only a ceaseless becoming; it is, and it is also not; and its comprehension is not so much a knowledge as an illusion.[10]

In Schopenhauer's view, both authors express the same basic idea: there is a difference between a world we perceive and a world lying 'beyond' this world-as-representation.[11] I return in Chapter 9 to Schopenhauer's interpretation of Plato's Ideas, which he embeds in his aesthetic theory.

Schopenhauer also claims that this dualism can be found in several Eastern scriptures: 'the same truth, though presented quite differently, is also a principal teaching of the *Vedas* and *Puranas*, namely the doctrine of Maya, by which is understood nothing but what Kant calls the phenomenon as opposed to the thing-in-itself'[12] (I will return to the concept of 'Maya' in Chapters 7 and 8). As briefly mentioned in Chapter 2, Schopenhauer also refers to Berkeley in this context, adding another rather different author to a group of thinkers that, in his view, all express the idea that 'whatever exists, exists only for the subject'.[13]

Again, as argued in Chapter 2, it remains unclear to what extent Schopenhauer believes the world-as-representation to really exist: whereas he at places argues that it *does* exist and that our perception of objects is based on sense data the subject receives from a material world in which it is firmly embedded as a corporeal being, he states in his most mystical passages that it is an illusion. In the following, we will see that his discussion of the world-as-will complicates this issue even more.

The inner being of phenomena

Following the dualisms developed by the above-mentioned authors, Schopenhauer claims that there is a world beyond or 'underneath' the world that we perceive: the world-as-will. The observation that the world we perceive is in some way or another dependent on, or at least structured by the perceiving subject, however, does not necessarily imply that we need to postulate a world 'beyond' the world-as-representation. This is where Schopenhauer introduces one of his most interesting arguments: whereas the body, as we have seen in Chapter 2, pulls his notion of the transcendental subject into the world-as-representation, it *also* plays a fundamental role in the world-as-will, forming 'a key to the inner being of every phenomenon in nature'.[14]

Schopenhauer defines this 'inner being' of phenomena in nature as 'Will', a concept that initially refers to an experience of our bodies that is not captured by anything described from the perspective of the world-as-representation, but that he eventually extrapolates to metaphysical claims about a world-as-will that forms the 'real' or 'true' essence of the world. In contrast with Kant, who attempts to say as little as possible about the in-itself, Schopenhauer thus claims that we have access to the 'absoluteness' Simmel mentions in the passage quoted above; that we can leap over the walls of the 'castle of the world-as-representation'[15] *through the body*. The corporeal dimension of our existence, in other words, provides a 'loophole' out of this world and a *key* to another world.

This idea is based on the following argument: what we experience inside of our bodies is fundamentally different from the organized and structured world in which I am a body-as-object in a world-of-objects – the world-as-representation – since I have an *intimate* and *direct* experience of my body that is different from my body as an object. This inner experience is my body experienced *as Will*:

> Something in the consciousness of everyone distinguishes the representation of his own body from all others that are in other respects

> quite like it. This is that the body occurs in consciousness in quite another way, *toto genere* different, that is denoted by the word will. It is just this double knowledge of our own body which gives us information about that body itself..., about what it is, not as representation, but as something over and above this, and hence what it is in itself. We do not have such immediate information about the nature, action, and suffering of any other real objects.[16]

Schopenhauer uses the rather confusing concept of 'Will', since it, in his view, approaches the experience he describes the closest: 'the concept of *will* is of all possible concepts the only one that has its origin *not* in the phenomenon, not in the mere representation of perception, but which comes from within, and proceeds from the most immediate consciousness of everyone.'[17]

Otherness

This 'Will', this 'direct contact' I have with my body that is different from the contact I have with objects around me, refers for Schopenhauer to a wide range of experiences. On one level, 'Will' captures the observation that I can move my body but that the nature of my bodily movements is not entirely clear to me. If I raise my arm, for example, this movement is different from someone else raising his or her arm since *I* raise *my* arm *as an agent*. However, the *exact* way in which I raise my arm remains unclear to me – I 'just raise it'. Willing myself to raise my arm and actually raising my arm is, within a certain understanding of 'willing', the same: 'actual willing is inseparable from doing, and, in the narrowest sense, that alone is an act of will which is stamped as such by the deed.'[18] It is this 'magical' or 'unexplainable' aspect of physical actions, their underlying unexplainable 'force' or 'energy', that Schopenhauer refers to with 'Will'.[19]

On another level, Schopenhauer refers with 'Will' to the impulses, desires and urges we experience as existing 'inside' of our bodies, like hunger, thirst, aggression or fear. Most famously, he refers here to the drive to self-preservation, portraying living creatures as consisting of a need to survive, an *ungraspable* but powerful 'force of life' that he sometimes describes as 'will-to-live' but also as drive to self-preservation: 'if we consider the will where no one denies it, namely in knowing beings, we find everywhere, as its fundamental effort, the *self-preservation* of every being: *Omnis natura vult esse conservatrix sui.*'[20]

Furthermore, Schopenhauer refers to sexual urges, going at places so far as claiming that they form the *kernel* of living beings: 'it is really the invisible central point of all action and conduct, and peeps up everywhere, in spite of all the veils thrown over it'.[21] He observes:

> The sexual impulse is the kernel of the will-to-live, and consequently the concentration of all willing.... Indeed, it may be said that man is concrete sexual impulse, for his origin is an act of copulation, and the desire of his desires is an act of copulation, and this impulse alone perpetuates and holds together the whole of his phenomenal appearance.... The sexual desire is the most vehement of cravings.... Accordingly, its satisfaction, corresponding exactly to the individual desire of anyone, thus to a desire directed to a definite individual, is the summit and crown of happiness, the ultimate goal of his natural endeavours.[22]

Schopenhauer herewith takes an enormously complex range of bodily and instinctive experiences – sexual desires, hunger, thirst, but also the ability to move – and groups them together under the concept of 'Will'.[23]

The first aspect that unites the range of experiences Schopenhauer categorizes under 'Will' is the idea that these experiences *as experiences* cannot be perceived from an external point of view; to put it in Schopenhauer's terms: they cannot be perceived 'in' the world-as-representation.[24]

Another general characteristic is the idea that the body-as-will is, to a certain extent, 'the other' of me. Again, this 'otherness' is understood in Schopenhauer's philosophy in a very general manner. It refers both to the 'mysterious' character of me moving my limbs while I do not consciously understand 'how' I exactly do this, and to the experience of, for example, sexual desires that at certain moments can cloud my rational thoughts and play a defining role in my deeds and actions. A part of this aura of 'otherness' is thus formed by the idea we are not able to fundamentally *explain* or *understand* these desires nor entirely *control* them.[25]

Metaphysical extrapolation

This brings us to Schopenhauer's metaphysics: whereas we see, taste, smell, hear and touch a world around us in which our bodies exist as individual objects, the experiencing self to which this world presents itself as phenomenon *also* experiences his or her own body-as-will. In turn, this Will is understood as so fundamentally 'other' *and* at times so fundamentally overpowering that Schopenhauer *extrapolates* this experience to a notion of what the world essentially is. In other words: we do not only, in Schopenhauer's view, *experience* ourselves as striving beings; he goes further and claims that our bodies are 'objectifications' or 'manifestations' of this striving and are therefore manifestations of something *transcending* us as individual bodies:

> The double knowledge which we have of the nature and action of our own body, and which is given in two completely different ways, has now been clearly brought out. Accordingly, we shall use it further as a key to the inner being of every phenomenon in nature. We shall judge all objects which are not our own body, and therefore are given to our consciousness not in a double way, but only as representations, according to the analogy of this body. We shall therefore assume that as, on the one hand, they are representation, just like our body, and are in this respect homogeneous with it, so on the other hand, if we set aside their existence as the subject's representation, what still remains over must be, according to its inner nature, the same as what in ourselves we call will.[26]

The *microcosm* that human beings are – experiencing themselves in two different ways – forms the basis for a metaphysical notion of the *macrocosm* that we, as microcosms, are part of. In Schopenhauer's words: 'everyone in this twofold regard is the whole world in itself, the microcosm; he finds its two sides whole and complete within himself';[27] 'every knowing individual is therefore in truth, and finds himself as, the whole will-to-live, or as the in-itself of the world itself, and also as the complimentary condition of the world as representation, consequently as a microcosm to be valued equally with the macrocosm.'[28]

This latter world – the world 'beyond' or 'below' the world-as-representation – is characterized by Schopenhauer as 'one', as not consisting of different objects or bodies but as a blind drive; a force that underlies everything there is, forming the 'inner' or 'true' core of the world we *perceive* as existing of separate phenomena. There are no individual things, objects or human beings 'in' the world-as-will; there is no *principium individuationis*, no time, space or causality since these are forms by which the subject perceives the world.

It is here that Schopenhauer arrives at his most mystical observations, inspired by Buddhism and Hinduism:

> The will as thing-in-itself is entire and undivided in every being, just as the centre is an integral part of every radius; whereas the peripheral

> end of this radius is in the most rapid revolution with the surface that represents time and its content, the other end at the centre where eternity lies, remains in profoundest peace, because the centre is the point whose rising half is no different from the sinking half.... Here, of course, we fall into mystical and metaphorical language, but it is the only language in which anything can be said about this wholly transcendent theme.[29]

Critics of Schopenhauer's metaphysics

An anthropologization of nature

This 'broadening' or 'extrapolating' of the experience of an *otherness* of a wide range of bodily experiences to the claim that there is a world-in-itself that is, to a certain extent, *like* these experiences within ourselves; this 'Sprung', as Volker Spierling calls it in his introduction to Schopenhauer's lectures on morality, 'vom psychologischen Willen zum Ding an sich, vom empirischen Standpunkt zum metaphysischen Standpunkt'[30] is highly problematic and has been subject to several critical attacks.[31]

In his famous essay 'The Bourgeois Irrationalism of Schopenhauer's Metaphysics', which I briefly mentioned in the Introduction to this book, Lukács argues, for example, that Schopenhauer relapses into an irrational celebration of mystical experiences that removes his philosophy entirely from the sphere of systematic and rational thought: 'Schopenhauer anthropologizes the whole of Nature with the help of plain analogy, which he loftily declares to be myth, and hence truth.[32] Lukács therefore deems Schopenhauer's philosophy to be based on pure 'sophistry'.[33]

A similar point is made by Adorno, who in *Negative Dialectics* characterizes the concept of 'Will' as an 'identity principle' that is 'borrowed from the idealistic system'.[34] Schopenhauer uses a concept, an idea originating in the mind and projects it onto the world as a whole, Adorno observes. Thereby, he subsumes everything that exists under a mental category. Instead of bringing us closer to the nature of the world, this means that Schopenhauer in fact brushes its otherness away and reduces it to a unifying subjective principle that originates in thought. A similar point was formulated by Nietzsche, who concluded that Schopenhauer's doctrine of the Will is a failure, permeated with contradictions.[35]

Another problematic aspect of Schopenhauer's discussion of 'Will', following from Lukács and Adorno's observations, is that it completely lacks a historical or culturally relativistic dimension: the desires and urges we experience within ourselves follow, in his view, from the metaphysical essence of the world. This makes Schopenhauer blind to the idea that many of our needs are influenced by the social and cultural norms and ideas surrounding us, that the way in which we experience our sexuality, for example, is permeated with the ideals and norms of our times and of the ways of thinking – religious, social, cultural, economic, political, educational – that we incorporate into our selves.[36]

From a historicist and psycho-social point of view, it could therefore even be argued that Schopenhauer's ideas about corporeality mirror a historical age and society in which the body is approached as an object of otherness that contrasts acutely with the rational mind, even enslaving it. In Chapter 7, I show that Adorno indeed interprets Schopenhauer's ideas on compassion and embodiment as neurotic responses to feelings of unfreedom that are portrayed as following from an unchangeable (inner and outer) nature.

Defence

Several attempts have been made to save Schopenhauer from this rather devastating critique. Regarding the idea that 'Will' is too broad a concept, for example, Bryan Magee argues that we should use the word 'force' instead of 'Will' in order to avoid any confusion with 'volition' or with the idea of a worldly purpose or goal. Magee's argument is based on Schopenhauer's rather totalizing claims that this 'Will' is present in both alive and lifeless entities in the world – from gravity to growing plants to human beings – making it into a physical and 'neutral' force instead of into anything related to the human will.[37]

Even though Schopenhauer indeed claims, at places, that 'forces' or 'natural laws' fall under the concept of 'Will' as well,[38] using the word 'force' only highlights the problematic nature of his extrapolation from microcosm to macrocosm: Schopenhauer, after all, starts with an analysis of the body, of movements, feelings and desires within this body that we do not entirely understand, and *then* broadens this observation to the claim that the natural 'forces' in the world around us are basically of the same nature. Using the concept of 'force' to refer to sexual desires and the drive to self-preservation, as Magee proposes, stretches these drives so far that their *specific* nature and their *specific* influence on human behaviour are lost. Schopenhauer claims, after all, that Will 'is infinitely better known and more intimate than anything else'.[39]

Georg Simmel develops yet another interpretation of 'Will', arguing as well that Schopenhauer's metaphysics is in danger of becoming a 'myth' or 'fantastic anthropomorphism'.[40] In contrast with Magee,

Simmel urges us to understand 'Will' as *still* belonging to the realm of phenomena: 'we do not touch the untouchable, but we approach it as closely as possible, stopping at a point which still is not the thing-in-itself but is only its clearest and most intimate revelation.'[41] We *experience* Will, which means, in Simmel's view, that what we experience must *remain* within the realm of the phenomenal, defining this idea as 'thinking about the absolute within the confines of the relative'.[42]

Again, however, this interpretation does not solve the problem: how can we say anything about being 'closer' to a metaphysical realm if we are unable to describe this realm? In what way is 'the impenetrable veil covering our absolute being the thinnest'?[43] And why are we justified in claiming that the metaphysical realm beyond our experience is *like* the way we experience Will within ourselves at all?

Schopenhauer's solutions

Schopenhauer himself does not offer us a convincing answer to these questions either. At some places he claims that through our bodies we have a *direct* access to the world-*in-itself* and that the Will we experience within ourselves is 'a narrow gateway to truth':[44] 'our willing is the only opportunity we have of understanding simultaneously from within any event that outwardly manifests itself; consequently it is the one thing known to us immediately, and not given to us merely in the representation, as all else is.'[45] In his lectures on *Metaphysik der Sitten* he even explicitly claims that the Will is 'das Wesen an sich im Menschen.'[46]

At other places, however, Schopenhauer urges us to understand that this 'immediate experience' does not mean that we experience the world-in-itself *as it really is*.[47] Although 'space' and 'causality' do not structure our knowledge of the Will, for example, the inner form of time does, in his view:

> There still remains the form of *time*, as that of being known and of knowing in general. Accordingly, in this inner knowledge the thing-in-itself has indeed to a great extent cast off its veils, but still does not appear quite naked. In consequence of the form of time, which still adheres to it, everyone knows his *will* only in its successive individual *acts*, not as a whole, in and by itself.[48]

Still, Schopenhauer here seems to argue, the world-in-itself is hidden behind a veil and there remains a difference between world-as-will and world-in-itself. In *On the Basis of Morality* he refers as well to a 'great and essential part that remains hidden from and unknown to everyone'.[49]

Schopenhauer makes this discussion even more unclear by suggesting, as briefly mentioned above, that human beings are *manifestations* of Will and thereby problematizes the question of what the exact content of the world we perceive is, discussed in Chapter 2. We experience strivings and desires, Schopenhauer claims, because we *are* metaphysical strivings and desires manifested *in* the world-as-representation. He argues in a peculiar passage:

> The parts of the body must correspond completely with the chief demands and desires by which the will manifests itself; they must be the visible expression of these desires. Teeth, gullet, and intestinal canal are objectified hunger; the genitals are objectified sexual impulse; grasping hands and nimble feet correspond to the more indirect strivings of the will which they represent.[50]

The above-mentioned paintings of Francis Bacon come to mind, depicting bodies torn apart by fear, anxiety and suffering, losing their specific shapes as understandable objects and turning into manifested suffering and lust, into almost unrecognizable matter torn apart by its own essence.

Trichotomy

One of the most helpful interpretations of (and struggles with) the relationship between world-as-will and world-in-itself in Schopenhauer's philosophy is developed by Julian Young in *Willing and Unwilling*. Young defends the idea that Schopenhauer's philosophy is based on a 'trichotomy' instead of on a dichotomy between *noumenon* and *phenomenon*. Within ourselves, he argues, we experience a world that is interposed 'between noumenal reality on the one hand and the ordinary world (the world as conceived by common sense and natural science ...) on the other, a third world distinct from either'.[51] This suggestion does justice to the notion that the world-as-will embodies an 'otherness' compared to the experiences we have of the world-as-representation, but also to the claim that it is *still* experienced by the self and therefore only *relatively* 'other':

> This third world, non-noumenal and hence situated within the Kantian boundaries, yet esoteric and so distinct from the ordinary world, could then constitute the topic of metaphysical investigation. And such an investigation could ... provide a genuinely extraordinary, exotic world-description worthy of the adjective 'metaphysical', were

> it the case that in constructing its world-description it made use of some aspect of experience neglected by our ordinary world-view (for example, inner experience of our wills) or, at least, extended the concept of the object of such experience radically beyond its usual sphere of application.[52]

Young's interpretation compromises many of Schopenhauer's claims and philosophical implications. Whereas Simmel could argue that the 'Will' within ourselves is a way of 'thinking about the absolute within the confines of the relative',[53] Young replaces the idea of an 'absolute' with the notion of a *feeling* of transcendence that nevertheless remains strictly within the confines of the relative. He understands 'Will' as a *dimension* of our experience that we cannot explain in ways in which we normally explain phenomena – this 'inexplicability' is what distinguishes it from the world-as-representation. However, any claims about a world-as-will lying beyond the regions of our experience are dismissed as too speculative and unjustified. Herewith, he partly does justice to the critique formulated by Lukács and Adorno, even though the ahistorical nature of Will is not addressed by his interpretation.

In light of the observation that we *either* have to pull the 'Will' close to our own experience *or* 'sanitize' it into a natural force, I believe Young's suggestion is quite convincing. Schopenhauer, after all, extrapolates from an individual experience to claims about the nature of the universe, not the other way around. Furthermore, even though he is rather unclear about what he precisely means, Schopenhauer himself often pointed in this same direction: Spierling quotes a passage from a letter written by Schopenhauer in 1852 claiming that his philosophy does not speak of '*Wolkenkukkuksheim*' ('cloud cuckoo land') but of '*dieser Welt*' – that he does not speak of metaphysical 'mumbo jumbo' or build castles in the air (of which he infamously accused Hegel) but that he refers to *this* world. In this letter, Schopenhauer also explicitly argues that he does not seek to write about the world-in-itself since every experience, everything we feel or notice 'within us' is always *already* a 'for us'. Schopenhauer thus states about his claim that the 'Will' is a key to the world-in-itself and forms the *Ding an sich* or thing-in-itself: 'Dieses aber ist Ding an sich blos relativ, d.h. in seinem Verhältniß zur Erscheinung: – und diese ist Erscheinung bloß in ihrer Relation zum ding an sich. Außerdem ist sie ein Gehirnphänomen. Was aber das Ding an sich außerhalb jener Relation sei, habe ich nie gesagt, weil ich's nicht weiß.'[54]

Compassion and Will

In the following, I want to build further upon Young's interpretation of Schopenhauer's metaphysics by highlighting what I see as its most interesting aspect: its role as the basis of a moral philosophy that revolves around compassion. Even though I agree with Adorno that Schopenhauer's concept of 'Will' is too speculative to be taken seriously as a consistent philosophical notion, following too obviously from an analysis of a bodily feeling of otherness that is transformed into a mental concept that is, in turn, projected onto the world as a whole, I herewith want to show that Schopenhauer's emphasis on compassion does highlight an interesting and unique aspect of embodiment.

The metaphysical basis of *Mitleid*

In *On the Will in Nature*, Schopenhauer argues that 'the only Metaphysics which really and immediately supports Ethics, is that one which is itself primarily ethical and constituted out of the material of Ethics'.[55] The reason why his metaphysic is 'constituted out of the material of Ethics' is found in the concept of *Mitleid*, which E.F.J. Payne translates as 'compassion' in his standard translation of Schopenhauer's chief work.[56]

Schopenhauer defines 'compassion' as 'the empirical appearance of the will's metaphysical identity, through the physical multiplicity of its phenomena';[57] an identity that is 'entirely different from that which is brought about by the forms of the phenomenon'.[58] He uses the word 'mysterious' in this context as well, providing the following phenomenological description of compassion:

> I no longer look at him [the suffering other] as if he were something given to me by empirical intuitive perception, as something strange and foreign, as a matter of indifference, as something entirely different from me. On the contrary, I share the suffering *in him*, in spite of the fact that his skin does not enclose my nerves. Only in this way can *his* woe, *his* distress, become a motive *for me*; otherwise it can be absolutely my own. I repeat that this *occurrence is mysterious*, for it is something our faculty of reason can give no direct account of, and its grounds cannot be discovered on the path of experience.[59]

It is important to stress that Schopenhauer argues that actions based on compassion, aimed at easing the pain or suffering of others, are *spontaneous* in nature: 'on the spur of the moment, without much reflection, one man helps another, helps to the assistance of one whom he has seen for the first time'.[60] As occurrences *that* short, impulses of compassion do not (yet) form part of conscious reflection, Schopenhauer claims, whereby he explicitly criticizes the idea (as formulated in Ubaldo Cassina's 1788 work *Saggio Analitico sulla Compassione*) that this phenomenon is based on *imagining* oneself to 'feel' the pains of the other 'in' oneself.[61]

We have to look at the supplement to *On the Basis of Morality* to understand the connection between this discussion and Schopenhauer's metaphysics. In this supplement, Schopenhauer describes the 'metaphysical foundation' of this 'mysterious' occurrence of compassion. This foundation brings us back to his ideas regarding the double knowledge we have of our bodies, described above:[62]

> [I]f plurality and separateness belong only to the *phenomenon*, and if it is one and the same essence manifests itself in all living things, then that conception that abolishes the difference between ego and non-ego is not erroneous; but on the contrary, the opposite conception must be.... Accordingly, it would be the metaphysical basis of ethics and consists in *one* individual's again recognizing in *another* his own true self, his own true inner nature.[63]

The phenomenon of compassion is understood as recognizing something of ourselves 'in the other' and therefore as the 'proper expression'[64] of the view that we are, on a fundamental level, 'connected' to other creatures:

> The barrier between the ego and non-ego is for the moment abolished; only then do the other man's affairs, his need, distress, and suffering directly become my own. I no longer look at him as if he were something given to me by empirical intuitive perception, as something strange and foreign, as a matter of indifference, as something entirely different from me. On the contrary, I share the suffering in him, in spite of the fact that his skin does not enclose my nerves.[65]

Furthermore, its occurrence, of which Schopenhauer claims that it is not bound to the sphere of reflection, implies that this 'recognizing' takes place on a corporeal level and precedes the world of distinctive objects and individuals that we perceive – the world-as-representation: 'beyond all plurality and diversity of individuals presented to us by the *principium individuationis,* there is to be found their unity.'[66] Someone who hurts another being, he claims, has not opened his or her eyes to the observation that he or she is like the mythological Thyestes: 'eagerly devouring his own flesh'.[67]

With these observations, we arrive at what I understand as the most interesting aspect of Schopenhauer's metaphysics: the body and its ability to experience both compassion and pain unite us, in his view, with each other on a level that transcends all other levels of existence.[68] He herewith develops a notion of connectedness that is fascinating because it is so radical in its egalitarian nature.[69]

Even though this idea follows from a metaphysics that Lukács characterizes as pure 'sophistry'[70] – we have seen above that many of Schopenhauer's metaphysical claims indeed are highly speculative and not very convincing[71] – Schopenhauer here infuses his idealism with naturalistic and materialistic ideas in a way that powerfully highlights an important dimension of human existence.

Mysticism and corporeality

As is the case with many of his claims, Schopenhauer is not entirely clear about the nature of compassion and in places clearly contradicts himself. In 'Compassion and Solidarity with Sufferers: the Metaphysics of *Mitleid*', David E. Cartwright provides an interesting analysis of the vagueness surrounding Schopenhauer's metaphysical notion of 'Will' and his understanding of what happens when we feel 'with' or 'in' the suffering of others. Cartwright shows that Schopenhauer sometimes argues that 'compassionate agents participate immediately in another's suffering',[72] implying that *intuitively* one feels the pain of another person *in* the other, recognizing one's self in the suffering person one perceives and thereby still holding on to a notion of 'self'. At other places, however, Schopenhauer argues that we are all 'one' on a metaphysical level, completely abandoning the idea of a self and focusing on an underlying and selfless 'unity of being'. Schopenhauer indeed even mentions the 'Mahāvākya' ('great saying') of the *Chāndogya Upanishad – 'Tat tvam asi'* or '*This art thou*' – to illustrate his idea that individuals form part of the same 'undivided whole'.[73]

Mystical claims like these, of course, conflict rather acutely with the observation that we do not feel compassion with suffering persons whom we do not perceive or about whom we do not know. To put it in Schopenhauer's terms: there has to be some sort of connection to suffering others through the world-as-representation in order to feel compassion with them.[74] Another important observation that conflicts with the metaphysical status Schopenhauer provides to the phenomenon of compassion is that in many cases people *fail* to display compassion towards each other. I return to this latter issue in Chapter 4.

Following these observations and Young's suggestion described above, I believe that the most convincing aspects of Schopenhauer's analysis of compassion are those formulated within a phenomenological and less metaphysical framework, referring to 'pre-individualistic' and 'direct' feelings that are nevertheless experienced *within* the body. In places, these aspects border on the naturalistic: Schopenhauer even refers to non-human animals as capable of experiencing compassion for each other, and to human beings 'feeling with' the suffering of non-human animals:[75]

> The moral incentive advanced by me as the genuine, is further confirmed by the fact that the animals are also taken under its protection. In other European systems of morality they are badly provided for, which is most inexcusable.... In philosophy it rests, despite all evidence to the contrary, on the assumed total difference between man and animal.[76]

Schopenhauer hereby extends morality to the animal world, criticizing 'Western forms of philosophy' (as opposed to Eastern traditions) for creating a 'vast chasm, an immeasurable gulf between man and animal in order to represent them as fundamentally different'.[77] I return to this issue in Chapter 7.

Conclusion

We have seen that, as is the case with his epistemology, the body plays a prominent role in Schopenhauer's metaphysics: our corporeality forms the key to the world-as-will, representing an ungraspable 'otherness' to a world governed by laws and defined by the *principium individuationis* – the world-as-representation. We have also seen that his metaphysical system contains several problematic contradictions and paradoxes. Whereas Schopenhauer in places argues that our bodies provide us with a direct experience of the in-itself, in his more convincing passages he refers to the phenomenological nature of an experience of striving and otherness within our bodies.

Furthermore, even though he approaches the world-as-representation as completely different from the world-as-will, Schopenhauer keeps pulling these two worlds together by placing both in the realm of human experience, and more specifically, within the realm of *bodily* experience. Thereby his desire to do justice to naturalistic observations regarding the body – not just as a perceiving entity but also as a striving and desiring being – forces him to breach the gap between *noumenon* and *phenomenon*, the body forming the bridge crossing this gap. Whereas he argues that the world-as-representation is experienced by a body with sense organs that exists within this same world, he observes that the world-as-will is experienced within a striving and desiring body that allows us to 'connect' to other people on an instinctive level, transcending our individual bodies and, through this process, experiencing compassion. However, he implies that even this striving, metaphysical body is part of the world-as-representation: Schopenhauer argues, after all, that our bodies are manifestations of Will *in* the world-as-representation, thereby clearly connecting both worlds: 'the whole body must be nothing but my will become visible, must be my will itself.'[78]

Even though I have argued that this metaphysical system is deeply flawed, I have also tried to show that Schopenhauer's discussion of the world-as-will follows from an interesting approach to human existence that emphasizes corporeality. Following our analysis of both his understanding of the world-as-representation and world-as-will, we can therefore conclude that Schopenhauer tries to develop a form of idealism in which the body plays such a prominent role that it eventually pushes the mind from its pedestal. Regarding his analyses of both worlds, I have therefore argued that his most convincing observations and arguments are those following from a phenomenological approach to the embodied subject. By adopting this phenomenological approach, the idealistic system Schopenhauer constructs (and thereby the dualism between *noumenon* and *phenomenon*) slowly crumbles down and transforms into a peculiar form of metaphysical materialism that revolves around two different ways in which the embodied subject relates to the world in which it lives.

4
Irrationalism and Pessimism

Introduction

The *oeuvre* of the Japanese author Yukio Mishima revolves for an important part around the corporeal dimension of human existence and the struggles the writer experienced with and within his body. He criticized the idea that the body and its 'language' can entirely be captured or subsumed by the world of ideas or by rational thought and understood the firmness, strength and *otherness* of corporeality as an antipode to the world of the mind:

> Why should the area of the skin, which guarantees a human being's existence in space, be most despised and left to the tender mercies of the senses? I could not understand the laws governing the motion of thought – the way it was liable to get stuck in unseen chasms whenever it is set out to go deep; or, whenever it aimed at heights, to soar away into boundless and equally invisible heavens, leaving the corporeal form undeservedly neglected.[1]

Mishima also understood his body as the cause of his melancholia; he struggled with his sexual feelings and with the realization that the body changes and eventually dies. In this context Schopenhauer observes: 'just as we know our walking to be only a constantly prevented falling, so is the life of our body only a constantly prevented dying, an ever-deferred death.'[2] By way of bodybuilding Mishima tried to fight this 'constant falling': 'the body is doomed to decay, just like the complicated motor of a car. I for one do not, will not, accept such a doom. This means that I do not accept the course of Nature.'[3]

Mishima understood his existence as consisting of a tension between *body* on the one hand and *consciousness* on the other; between *instincts* and *self-reflection*; between *flesh* and *thought-world*; between 'Ideas' and 'Nature'. He furthermore argued that this tension becomes most apparent in experiences of pain and suffering,[4] implying that the body is independent of ideas and cultural and social influences.

Mishima's observations on the body resulted in his idea that human beings are a paradox of existence, a 'form of existence that rejects existence'.[5] In his view, humans are irrational, natural and impulsive creatures that are able to rationally reflect on their situation *as* natural, impulsive creatures but, at the same time, cannot escape the impulsive and striving body, nor the fact that this body decays and eventually dies.

This brings us to the topic of this chapter, in which I will look at the consequences of Schopenhauer's hitherto discussed analyses of the world-as-representation and the world-as-will for his pessimistic understanding of the human condition. The idea that human beings are characterized by a tension between the irrational body and the rational mind will play a central role in this analysis. I will argue that, in Schopenhauer's view, human beings are enslaved by their bodies and have no rational control over their fate and that, like in the case of Mishima, this idea resulted in his pessimism.

We herewith also arrive at one of the most-formulated points of critique against Schopenhauer, which are aimed at his idea that if we have no rational control over our bodies or over the world, then we are completely helpless, doomed to accept our fate in an irrational and chaotic world and to dismiss the faculty of reason as powerless and useless. Popper famously characterized Schopenhauer as 'the father of modern irrationalism'[6] and, as mentioned in the Introduction to this book, Lukács argued in 'The Bourgeois Irrationalism of Schopenhauer's Metaphysics' that Schopenhauer defends a 'reactionary mysticism' that is blind to the realities of history and human existence and pessimistically accepts the horrors of the world by refusing to accept the idea that as rational beings we can influence and change the world in which we live. As the title of his essay suggests, an important part of Lukács' critique indeed revolves around the idea that there is no room for rational and autonomous action in Schopenhauer's philosophy: 'with Schopenhauer we are dealing with inwardness pure and simple, with the philosophical and ethical devaluation of every action, every real deed.'[7]

In order to evaluate this 'charge of irrationalism', we first need to define precisely what is meant by the concept of 'irrationality'. In this chapter, I will do this by following Julian Young's helpful essay 'Is Schopenhauer an Irrationalist?', in which it is argued that this 'charge' can be divided into three different claims regarding three different kinds of irrationalism: ontological, epistemological and practical. I will link these three forms of irrationalism to three aspects of Schopenhauer's pessimism by developing the argument that Schopenhauer's ideas on the irrational nature of both world and body form the basis of his infamous pessimistic diagnosis of the human condition.

Ontological irrationalism

A blind universe

The first kind of irrationalism Young discerns is *ontological* in nature: being an ontological irrationalist implies that one categorically denies what Young calls 'the isomorphism of reason and reality'.[8] An ontological irrationalist claims that reality is not structured in a rational or logical sense and argues that we are 'profoundly *not* at home in the world'.[9] Characterizing Plato as an ontological rationalist, Young claims that Nietzsche is his 'paradigmatic antagonist'.[10]

Young rightfully concludes that Schopenhauer belongs to the Nietzschean end of this spectrum:[11] as we have seen in Chapter 3, Schopenhauer's metaphysical doctrine denies the idea that the essence of the world is structured rationally or mirrors the rational mind. The universe consists of a Will Schopenhauer defines as 'blind', after all, a striving that has no purpose or goal and that goes on endlessly without resolve.

With this observation we arrive at Schopenhauer's first argument for pessimism: if the world essentially consists of blind striving and has no purpose, and if this striving is understood as the essence of the universe and, hence, as something over which we have no control, then we are born in a world that is devoid of meaning, purpose or sense. As discussed in the Introduction, Schopenhauer indeed inverts Leibniz' famous dictum into the observation that 'a worse world could not continue to exist, it is absolutely impossible; and so this world itself is the worst of all possible worlds'.[12]

Not only does Schopenhauer herewith break with most religious traditions, he also breaks with any philosophical system that claims that the world or human history develop towards a goal, progress towards a better state or are organized in light of a greater purpose.

Striving and desiring

Schopenhauer's ontological irrationalism also has severe consequences for his ideas on embodiment: if the world consists of irrational striving and if our bodies are manifestations of this same irrational striving, then the irrational nature of the world is mirrored by the irrationality of our bodies. Not only are we not at home in the world, Schopenhauer's philosophy herewith suggests, we are also not at home in our own bodies.

In Chapter 3 we have seen that Schopenhauer argues that human beings are manifestations of 'Will', of the endless striving that is the essence of the universe. As bodily creatures, manifestations of Will, we constantly desire, want and need, he claims, and when one desire is satisfied we experience a brief moment of emptiness and boredom before the next desire arises, resulting in a miserable existence consisting of a constant dependency on the satisfaction of our needs. Famously, he therefore states that human life 'swings like a pendulum to and fro between pain and boredom'[13] and observes:

> Far from bearing the character of a *gift*, human existence has entirely the character of a contracted *debt*. The calling in of this debt appears in the shape of the urgent needs, tormenting desires, and endless misery brought about through that existence. As a rule, the whole lifetime is used for paying off this debt, yet in this way only the interest is cleared off. Repayment of the capital takes place through death.[14]

But Schopenhauer goes even further, characterizing human existence as a 'mistake' and death as the logical undoing of this mistake: 'Death ... is the violent destruction, bursting in from outside, of the fundamental error of our true nature, the great disillusionment. At bottom, we are something that ought not to be; therefore we cease to be.'[15] Frequently, he therefore refers to Theognis' line that 'better not to be born at all would be the best thing for man, never to behold the sun's scorching rays.'[16] This means that our existence as corporeal creatures makes it impossible to find happiness, an observation that forms another argument for Schopenhauer's pessimism: 'Everything in life proclaims that earthly happiness is destined to be frustrated, or recognized as an illusion. The grounds for this lie deep in the very nature of things.'[17] 'There is only one inborn error', Schopenhauer indeed concludes, 'and that is the notion that we exist in order to be happy.'[18]

The main assumption behind these claims is that it is an entirely *negative* experience to feel irrational desires, which follows from Schopenhauer's understanding of the specific nature of the strivings that engulf us. Not only can they not be satisfied and therefore provide us with a permanent experience of restlessness, they also 'flow through' us as individual bodies, as it were, and give us the experience of 'bursting out of our skin', his metaphysical system suggests.

Furthermore, Schopenhauer argues that happiness itself is 'negative' in nature: it consists of an *absence* of a state of striving instead of a *presence* of certain feelings.[19] He writes: 'We feel pain, but not painlessness; care, but not freedom from care; fear, but not safety and security. We feel the desire as we feel hunger and thirst; but as soon as it has been satisfied, it is like the mouthful of food that has been taken, and which seizes to exist for our feelings the moment it has been swallowed.'[20] Within Schopenhauer's philosophy, in other words, it is not possible to experience striving or desiring in a positive manner: we are driven from desire to satisfaction by a 'painful hollowness'[21] that needs to be filled, but once it is filled we merely experience boredom.

This idea is not very convincing: following Theognis' line that 'better not to be born at all would be the best thing for man, never to behold the sun's scorching rays',[22] we could argue, for example, that the feeling of the warmth of the sun on our skin can be a very pleasurable experience that does not just consist of an absence of suffering. The same can be said about sexual love and the satisfaction it may give us: even though this satisfaction does not last forever and, indeed, new desires may 'present themselves' to us later, this does not necessarily mean that satisfying these desires cannot be a very intimate, warm and happy experience. In fact, it may actually be the temporary nature of these experiences that makes them unique and pleasurable. This latter idea returns in Adorno's understanding of happiness, which I discuss in Chapter 10.

Pain

Schopenhauer's idea that human beings essentially are manifestations of irrational striving has a second implication, which follows from his ontological irrationalism and provides his philosophy with a materialistic aura. This implication revolves around the phenomenon of pain, which Schopenhauer describes as follows: 'everything that obstructs, crosses or opposes our will, and thus everything unpleasant and painful, is felt by us immediately, at once, and very plainly',[23] and: 'pain concerns the *will* alone and consists in checking, hindering, or thwarting this.'[24] Since everything that opposes the Will causes us pain – Georg Simmel phrases this idea as follows: 'in reality, pain is but the rape of our will'[25] – the fact that we are bodily manifestations of an irrational Will implies that our corporeality makes us into beings that are vulnerable to pain and suffering.

Schopenhauer's ontological irrationalism, the idea that the world is not organized rationally and that we are therefore not 'at home' in this world, herewith finds another basis in the idea that we are born as bodies that are manifestations of an irrational striving, which makes us vulnerable to pain. Schopenhauer indeed mentions suffering as one of the key aspects of the human condition and frequently refers to pain to develop a diagnosis of the state of the world as a whole. He argues in a famous passage: 'whoever wants summarily to test the assertion that the pleasure in the world outweighs the pain, or at any rate that the two balance each other, should compare the feelings of an animal that is devouring another with those of that other.'[26] Pain and suffering form the core of most of his observations on human existence and are understood by him as one of our most intimate forms of contact with the Will.

This means that we not only feel not at home in the world since this world is not organized rationally and since our bodies torment us with irrational and unstoppable desires, but also because our bodies make us vulnerable to pain. The nature of both world and body, Schopenhauer suggests, undermines the possibility of finding happiness.

Epistemological irrationalism

The external world

According to Young, a second way in which we can understand the 'charge of irrationalism' is in epistemological terms. He defines epistemological rationalism as the doctrine that 'the character of ultimate reality is accessible to us through, uniquely, the faculty of reason'.[27] We have seen in Chapters 2 and 3 that Schopenhauer claims that we have two forms of access to the world in which we live: through our perceptual apparatus, which constitutes the world-as-representation, and through our bodies, which form a key to the metaphysical kernel of the world. Both of these 'channels', he argues, are not rationally structured: we have seen that he infuses the framework he took over from Kant with naturalistic observations and argues, for example, that non-human animals experience the world-as-representation as well. Furthermore, he claims that the world-as-will is irrational, as is our access to it – through bodily feelings and desires. Both worlds, in other words, are described mainly from a phenomenological point of view in which the faculty of reason does not play a constitutive role.

Young argues, however, that Schopenhauer comes closer to rationalism than we might think because he arrives at an understanding of the world-as-will by way of rational argumentation. This argumentation, Young claims, can be found in *On the Fourfold Root of the Principle of Sufficient Reason,* in which Schopenhauer argues that we can define and describe the limits of our perceptual apparatus in a rational manner, which means that he does not 'simply' and uncritically embrace an irrational experience of the world.[28]

Young's analysis, however, is only partly convincing: even though it is true, as we have seen in Chapter 3, that Schopenhauer *argues* that the metaphysical *in-itself* of the world must be characterized by an absence of space, time and causality, he goes much further than Kant. Unlike the latter, he does not seek to describe the limits of our perceptual apparatus by concluding that we cannot say anything about the *in-itself,* but relies heavily on references to bodily experiences of 'otherness' to ground his descriptions of the metaphysical essence of the world. Most of his descriptions of Will, after all, follow from analyses of sexual desires, of hunger, of pain and of boredom. These references to bodily feelings are phenomenological in nature and have, in Schopenhauer's view, nothing to do with the faculty of reason. Another important observation is that the fact that Schopenhauer rationally analyses these experiences in his philosophical texts does not mean that our access to the world is *itself* rational in nature, as epistemological rationalists argue.

In Chapter 9, furthermore, I discuss Schopenhauer's understanding of an 'intuitive knowledge' of the world, which the subject gains once it reaches a state of salvation. We will see that this form of knowledge is not rational, logical or conceptual in nature either. Taking these observations into account, it is therefore rather difficult to argue that Schopenhauer is an epistemological rationalist.

The internal world

It is true, however, that Schopenhauer values the ability to rationally reflect and analyse the nature of the world. This is especially the case regarding his observations on the insight we are able to develop into our *own* nature. In order to evaluate Schopenhauer's understanding of rationality and the charge that he is an epistemological irrationalist, it is crucial to emphasize this latter aspect of his thought.

In order to analyse Schopenhauer's understanding of rational self-reflection, I want to look at a very important but often overlooked passage on freedom in the first volume of his chief work. In this passage, Schopenhauer explicitly refers to 'the deliberation of the faculty of reason' as follows:

> The possibility of ... freedom ... is man's greatest prerogative, which is for ever wanting in the animal, because the condition for it is the deliberation of the faculty of reason, enabling him to survey the whole of life independently of the impression of the present moment. ... Therefore the hungry wolf buries its teeth in the flesh of the deer with the same necessity with which the stone falls to the ground, without the possibility of the knowledge that it is the mauled as well as the mauler.[29]

What makes this specific passage interesting is that Schopenhauer here praises our ability to reflect on ourselves, which provides us, in his view, with *rational insight* into our existence as individuals – the insight that we are 'mauled as well as maulers'; that we are manifestations of something over which we have no control.

To a certain extent, this rational insight forms the driving force behind most of Schopenhauer's observations: like the theories of the three 'masters of suspicion' (to use Ricoeur's famous characterization) – Nietzsche, Marx, Freud[30] – his theory about the Will revolves around the idea that things are not what they seem; that below the surface of human behaviour a world is hidden, a realm of drives, instincts and mechanisms that steer our actions and ideals. With his philosophy, Schopenhauer seeks to unmask these actions and ideals, rid them of the positive and illusory aura we have provided them with and show what human life is really about.

An example can be found in Schopenhauer's analysis of sexuality. As briefly discussed in Chapter 2, he transforms his observations regarding the overpowering nature of Will into a theory that comes close to naturalistic and biological explanations of our sexual instincts as following from the struggle for the survival of our species. This makes individuals, Schopenhauer argues, into mere cogs in an overpowering machine that they have little to no control over: 'without knowing it, the individual here acts by order of something higher, the species'.[31]

Schopenhauer seeks to unmask the 'deep, unconscious seriousness' with which people who fall in love 'scrutinize each other' as in essence steered by the need to produce children that are as well-equipped for survival as possible.[32] In detail, he describes the physiological characteristics that people feel attracted to in their partners, reducing feelings of love and desire to physiological processes in the brain that make the idea of romantic love into a mere 'delusion'; a physiological 'trick' that, in turn, is a manifestations of a deeper lying striving that can only be understood as an affirmation of one's species as a whole:[33] 'while the lovers speak pathetically of the harmony of their souls, the core of the matter is often the agreement ... with regard to the being that is to be produced and to its perfection'.[34] He therefore concludes that 'all amorousness is rooted in the sexual impulse alone.'[35]

Another example is Schopenhauer's explanation of evil, of the need to purposely inflict pain and suffering on others. He argues that this phenomenon is the result of an intensification of the pathological state that human beings are always already in as manifestations of Will. A person committing evil deeds, he writes, is 'filled with an extremely intense pressure of will', tormented by 'terrible pain', 'frightful desolation' and 'emptiness'. This person keeps experiencing a drive within himself that has no 'recognized motive' and cannot be satisfied: 'he then seeks indirectly the alleviation of which he is incapable directly ..., he tries to mitigate his own suffering by the sight of another's, and at the same time recognizes this as an expression of his power. The suffering of another becomes for him an end in itself.'[36]

This affirmation of the ability to reflect on ourselves as rational creatures, however, does not result in a more positive understanding of humanity. Schopenhauer observes that rational insight enables us to realize that we are slaves, but does not provide us with the ability to break free from this situation.

Rationality as autonomy

Reflective endorsement

The idea that that we do not have control over our situation brings us to a third understanding of the 'charge of irrationalism': as implying that the ideas of rational self-constitution and of human freedom are illusions because human beings are ultimately driven by an irrational 'core' and are unable to rationally determine the ends of their actions. Young observes: 'it is ... [Schopenhauer's] views on human action and motivation which have ... figured most prominently as grounds for the charge [of irrationality].'[37]

Before evaluating the critical observation that Schopenhauer defends irrationality regarding human autonomy, I first want to develop a definition of the idea of a rational subject. A fascinating and influential understanding of what rationality implies has recently been developed by Christine Korsgaard, whose theory I want to discuss briefly to confront it with Schopenhauer's understanding of the faculty of reason. Furthermore, Korsgaard's theory returns in Chapter 8, in the context of an analysis of the role that the normativity of our bodily responses to pain and suffering plays in Schopenhauer's moral philosophy.

Starting from a broadly Kantian framework, Korsgaard argues that our ability to reflect on ourselves has created what she calls a 'reflective gap' between self-consciousness on the one hand and our 'nature' on the other hand. This gap forces us, she argues, to construct rational grounds for our actions:

> As I understand it, reason is a power we have in virtue of a certain type of self-consciousness – consciousness of the grounds of our own beliefs and actions. This form of self-consciousness gives us a capacity to control and direct our beliefs and actions that other animals lack, and make us active in a way that they are not. But it also gives us a problem that the other animals do not face – the problem of deciding what to count as a reason for belief or action.... The distinctive feature of human beings, reason, is therefore the capacity for normative self-government.[38]

Reason elevates us out of nature, in Korsgaard's view, because it enables us to put everything that we are into question. In *Primates and Philosophers: How Morality Evolved* she therefore argues against Dutch biologist Frans de Waal that what makes human beings fundamentally different from animals is the following capacity: 'we do not merely have intentions, good or bad. We assess and adopt them. We have the capacity for normative self-government, or, as Kant called it, "autonomy". It is at this level that morality emerges. The morality of your action is not a function of the content of your intentions. It is a function of the exercise of normative self-government.'[39]

Korsgaard herewith understands the birth of consciousness as originating in a dualism between self-reflection on the one hand and 'instinctual nature' on the other. She links this idea – with reference to Kant's interpretation of this biblical passage in *Conjectures on the Beginning of Human History* – to the allegory of the expulsion from the garden of Eden: 'our liberation from the government of instinct is also our expulsion from the Garden, our banishment from a world that is teleologically ordered by our instincts.'[40] Furthermore, Korsgaard argues, the 'reflective gap' between self-consciousness and nature forces us to argue *why* we should adopt certain norms or maxims as grounds for our actions and reject others: 'Each impulse as it offers itself to the will must pass a kind of test for normativity before we can adopt it as a reason for action.'[41] This results in her famous doctrine of *reflective endorsement*: 'the reflective mind must endorse the desire before it can act on it, it must say to itself that the desire is a reason.'[42]

Of course there is much more to Korsgaard's theory than I can discuss here. What I mainly want to show with this brief description of her theory is that there is a difference between acting *for a reason* and acting *in light of reason*: whereas the first kind of action is 'merely' based on *a* reason – for example: I reach for an apple because I am hungry and want to eat – the second kind of action is based on a rational evaluation of the grounds that present themselves to me as a conscious being, a process that ends with me deciding which ground I adopt as a *good* reason. In other words: whereas the first kind of behaviour can be characterized as 'rational' only in an *instrumental* sense, the second kind is rational in a *moral* manner and is uniquely linked to human existence; it revolves around the way in which I *decide* what kind of behaviour I want to adopt as a rational and reflective being and, furthermore, about the manner in which I thereby consciously seek to define myself as an autonomous person, *responsible* for my actions and deeds.

We can put the difference between these two kinds of rationality into words in yet another way, linking them to the notion of 'ends'. Whereas a person who acts rationally in an instrumental way merely seeks the best means to achieve an end that has not been selected rationally *itself* – for example, because that end follows from his or her 'nature' or biology – someone who acts rationally in the Korsgaardian sense of the term seeks to achieve an end that has *itself* been selected according to a rational procedure.

Empirical and intelligible characters

This brings us back to Schopenhauer who, like Korsgaard, grounds his analysis of freedom in Kant's ideas on autonomy. Unlike Korsgaard, however, he criticizes Kant's system for not being consistent and arrives at a radically different conclusion regarding the freedom of the rational self. He thereby specifically targets Kant's analysis of practical and transcendental freedom and his notions of the intelligible and the empirical character. In order to discuss Schopenhauer's ideas on freedom, I therefore first need to provide a short overview of these notions. I will thereby only sketch the contours of Kant's understanding of freedom. Furthermore, the scope of this chapter does not allow me to argue how Kant may be defended against Schopenhauer's critique: I am strictly concerned with the latter's understanding of freedom and determinism.

With practical freedom, Kant famously refers to the independence of our will from impulses of sensibility. This idea that can be proved through experience, he argues: we can observe that we are able to decide *not* to do something that our senses prompt us to do, he writes.[43] Transcendental freedom, Kant goes on, concerns the *possibility* of our making rational decisions as well as the radical initiation of an act. This initiation is *not* sensuous or bodily in nature, but is made possible by postulating a world fundamentally different from the empirical one: the *intelligible world*. This latter world cannot be known, since our knowledge is restricted to the empirical world, but we can nevertheless *conceive* of it in pure thought – a conception that makes it possible to attribute the freedom to determine the will to rational beings and therefore to conceive of rational beings as autonomous creatures, fully responsible for their actions: 'Without this freedom ... no moral law and no moral imputation are possible.'[44]

This brings us to Kant's understanding of the practical and the intelligible characters, concepts that Schopenhauer takes over but interprets in a radically different manner. In *Critique of Pure Reason* Kant describes the empirical character as follows:

> In virtue of its empirical character, [the] subject would ... be subordinate to all the empirical laws of causality, and, as a phenomenon and member of the sensuous world, its effects would have to be accounted for by a reference to preceding phenomena. External phenomena must be capable of influencing it; and its actions, in accordance with natural laws, must explain to us how its empirical character, that is, the law of its causality, is to be cognized in and by means of experience.[45]

If we observe a person 'from the outside', Kant thus claims, the notion of freedom does not present itself: in this light, every human being forms part of a chain of cause and effect and any movement that person makes, including its actions, are part of that same chain and therefore pre-determined.

Looking at him- or herself 'from the inside', Kant argues, a person appears to him- or herself in an altogether different manner. In *Critique of Pure Reason* he writes:

> In virtue of its intelligible character ... the subject must be regarded as free from all sensuous influences, and from all phenomenal determination. Moreover, as nothing *happens* in this subject – for it is a

> *noumenon*, and there does not consequently exist in it any change, demanding the dynamical determination of time, and for the same reason no connection with phenomena as causes – this active existence must in its actions be free from and independent of natural necessity, for this necessity exists only in the world of phenomena. It would be quite correct to say, that it originates or begins its effects in the world of sense *from itself*.[46]

If we look at ourselves from this perspective, in other words, we are able to approach ourselves as 'purely intelligible objects' and assign ourselves to the above-mentioned 'intelligible world'. It is by way of this non-empirical aspect of our being that Kant transcendentally guarantees the possibility of freedom.

The possibility of action

Schopenhauer's understanding of freedom and autonomy is based on a critique of this distinction between characters. Kant, Schopenhauer argues, made the mistake of trying to secure human freedom within a system that does not allow such a phenomenon to exist: the gap between the intelligible and the practical realms can, according to Kant's own theory, not be crossed since that would mean that a realm defined by freedom is linked to a realm permeated with causality.

The main problem with Kant's ideas on autonomy, Schopenhauer suggests, is that he equates will with reason, not realizing that the notion of will understood as a kind of spontaneity, as a force resulting in bodily movements, *has to* contain irrational, material and impulsive elements in order to be will *at all*. How can the intelligible character otherwise manifest itself as an active being in the practical realm? Holding true, in Schopenhauer's view, to Kant's original dichotomy, he claims that we have to conclude that the will has nothing whatsoever to do with reason: it belongs entirely to the empirical realm permeated with causality.

Schopenhauer puts this idea into words by referring to Kant's third antinomy, which consists of the *thesis*: 'Causality according to the laws of nature is not the only causality operating to originate the phenomena of the world. A causality of freedom is also necessary to account fully for these phenomena'; and the *antithesis*: 'There is no such thing as freedom, but everything in the world happens solely according to the laws of nature'.[47] Referring to this antinomy, Schopenhauer writes:

> In spite of all transcendental freedom..., no person has the capacity of himself to begin a series of actions, a thing which...was asserted by the thesis....Therefore right is entirely on the side of the antithesis;

> for this sticks to the point in question, and uses the principle of explanation which is valid in regard thereto; hence it needs no apology. The thesis, on the other hand, is supposed to be drawn by an apology from the matter that first passes over to something quite different from the point in question, and then takes over a principle of explanation which cannot be applied there.[48]

The only freedom we have, Schopenhauer argues, mainly in his essay 'On the Freedom of the Will' but also in *The World as Will and Representation*, is the freedom to do what we will. However, he goes on, the idea that we can decide *what* we will, that we can will to will something else, is an illusion. In other words, Schopenhauer answers the question of how the intelligible character can constitute an act, how 'pure consciousness' can cause an act in the empirical world, by stating that it cannot do this because reason has nothing to do with will and because a connection between the intelligible and the empirical realms cannot by definition, exist.

This notion of willing is based on a concept of the empirical character that he takes over from Kant but that Schopenhauer eventually uses in a completely different way. The empirical character, Schopenhauer argues, is the collection of qualities that make one into a specific person and, furthermore, that we can as well define as a person's will: since the self has no rational control over what it wills, there is no difference between willing and being and between willing and doing, Schopenhauer argues. Will and deed are the same: if someone would have wanted to do something different from what he or she is doing, this would have happened instead. In 'On the Freedom of the Will' Schopenhauer describes this idea as follows in a passage that is, like his analysis of the world-as-representation, influenced by naturalistic theories rising in his time:

> This particularly and individually constituted character of the will, by virtue of which its reaction to the same motives in every man is different, makes up that which one calls his character and, what is more, because it is not known a priori but only through experience, the empirical character. ... And, like the natural forces it too is original, unchangeable, and inexplicable. ... Only in the very highest, cleverest animals does a noticeable individual character manifest itself, although with the decisive preponderance of the species character.[49]

Acting, in other words, is self-expression according to Schopenhauer, an expression of that which one always *already* is: 'Man does at all times only what he wills, and yet he does this necessarily. But this is due to the fact that he already *is* what he wills. For from that which he *is*, there follows of necessity everything that he, at any time, *does*.'[50]

The freedom to act, Schopenhauer herewith concludes, is an illusion. Every being, as a bodily object, is embedded in a world defined by causality. And every bodily act, whether it is the reflex to pull one's hand away from something hot or the deliberate act of shaking someone's hand or writing down a sentence, forms part of a nexus of cause and effect, caused either by another event or triggered by one's empirical character, which is the 'empirically recognized, persistent, and unchangeable nature of an individual will'.[51]

Conceptual thought

It is crucial to notice that Schopenhauer does not ignore the capacity to think conceptually. He differentiates what he calls 'motives' from 'causes' (defining the movements of lifeless objects) and 'stimuli' (characterizing the movements of plants), and defines motivation as 'causality which passes through cognition'.[52] All animals can be motivated, he argues, which means that they are able to perceive something (for example, an apple), cognize this something (as an edible object), and then act (eat the apple). Unlike animals, furthermore, human beings are able to think conceptually and to form what Schopenhauer calls 'non-perceptual, abstract, general ideas' that can function as motives 'on' their empirical character.[53]

This does not mean, however, that human beings are free according to Schopenhauer. If someone has conflicting ideas, he claims, the following process takes place:

> The motives try out repeatedly, against one another, their effectiveness on the will. This puts the will in the same situation as that of the body on which different forces act in opposite directions, until finally the decidedly strongest motive drives the others from the field and determines the will. This outcome is called resolve, and it takes place with complete necessity.[54]

In other words: if we knew precisely a person's character and if we knew all the motives that presented themselves to this person (not just perceptions, but also thoughts, ideas and concepts), we would be able to predict what that person is going to do:

> Only in abstracto can several representations lie beside one another in consciousness as judgements and chains of conclusions, and then,

> free from all determination of time, work against one another, until the strongest overpowers the rest, and determines the will. This is the complete elective decision or faculty of deliberation which man has as an advantage over the animal, and on account of which freedom of will has been attributed to him, in the belief that his willing was a mere result of the operations of his intellect, without a definite tendency to serve at its basis. The truth is, however, that motivation works only on the basis and assumption of his definite tendency, that is in his case individual, in other words, a character.[55]

Atwell uses the word 'ground' to clarify what Schopenhauer means here: 'The character or will is simply the "ground" on which the operating motive causes the resultant action – this "ground" being necessary for any motive to operate, since motives alone or by themselves have no power.'[56] Schopenhauer himself uses the metaphor of a 'secret spring'.[57]

Even though the empirical character becomes apparent once we see more and more of what a person wills and does, Schopenhauer confusingly argues that the real basis of human behaviour is hidden from the conscious mind: we only know the ideas and concepts that occupy our thinking, as well as the feelings and emotions that we are conscious of. However, the main part of our character is 'hidden' or 'secret' and is defined by Schopenhauer as 'the dark recess of our inwardness'.[58] It thereby remains rather unclear where this 'inwardness' is located or how it is connected, on the one hand, to the world-as-representation in which it manifests itself as a causally active force, and on the other to the world-as-will to which it is, in some way or another, related as well. Acting, after all, exclusively happens in the world-as-representation, Schopenhauer repeatedly claims, and he therefore attempts to keep it away from any in-itself, Will or intelligible character that is not structured by causality. A person's will, in other words, can only play a role in the coming about of an act if this will is already manifested as a causally active force in the world-as-representation. But this raises the following questions: What is this will *before* it is manifested? And what is it a manifestation of precisely?

In places, Schopenhauer suggests that the empirical character should be understood as the 'temporal expression' of the intelligible character.[59] But this raises another question: how can we make sense of this 'expression' without referring to a *causal* connection between the intelligible character on the one hand and the world-as-representation on the other; in other words, without doing precisely that which Schopenhauer accuses Kant of? Like his ideas about the connection between the world-as-representation and the world-as-will (discussed in Chapter 3), according to which the latter 'manifests' itself as forces or desires 'in' the former, Schopenhauer's analysis of the connection between the intelligible and the empirical character remains highly problematic.

Even though he is unclear about these issues, it is important to notice that his observations strikingly anticipate the insights of psychoanalysis:[60]

> To make the matter clear, let us compare our consciousness to a sheet of water of some depth. Then the distinctly conscious ideas are merely the surface; on the other hand, the mass of the water is the indistinct, the feelings, the after-sensation of perceptions and intuitions and what is experienced in general, mingled with the disposition of our own will that is the kernel of our inner nature. Now this mass of the whole consciousness is more or less, in proportion to intellectual liveliness, in constant motion, and the clear pictures of the imagination, or the distinct, conscious ideas expressed in words, and the resolves of the will are what comes to the surface in consequence of this motion. The whole process of our thinking and resolving seldom lies on the surface, that is to say, seldom consists in a concatenation of clearly conceived judgements; although we aspire to this, in order to be able to give an account of it to ourselves and others.[61]

And he writes in another characteristic passage: 'Consciousness is the mere surface of our mind, and of this, as of the globe, we do not know the interior, but only the crust.'[62]

Since we are largely unaware of who we are and what decisions we will make, the notion of responsibility disappears in Schopenhauer's philosophy: our actions flow from a 'secret spring' over which we have no rational control. Schopenhauer, however, does develop an analysis of our *feelings* of responsibility. Since acts are 'symptoms' of our characters, he argues that we do not feel responsible for our acts, but for our *characters*. If we are tormented by guilt, he suggests, we do not wish we would have acted differently, but we wish we would have *been* differently; we wish we 'would have been someone else'.[63]

Determinism

In this paragraph I want to return to the question: in what sense can Schopenhauer be understood as an irrationalist? Even though the passages quoted above are rather clear about the idea that the ends of human behaviour are, in Schopenhauer's view, determined by an unknowable essence that human beings have no control over as rational and reflective creatures, in places he *does* seem to grant the rational self some power. He is unclear, however, about the manner in which those passages can be made compatible with his conclusions regarding the determined nature of the human animal.

One can find passages in his works in which he suggests that even abstract forms of deliberation and rational arguments are dependent on a person's will: 'In all abstract employment of the mind, the will is also the ruler. According to its intentions, the will imparts direction to the employment of the mind, and also fixes the attention',[64] and: 'knowing, and thus the intellect, presenting itself in self-consciousness wholly as the secondary element, is to be regarded not merely as the will's accident, but as its work; knowledge is thus by a roundabout way traceable again to the will.'[65]

At other places, however, he contradicts himself and writes: 'what bride and bit are to an unmanageable horse, the intellect is to the will in man; it must be led by the bridle by means of instruction, exhortation, training, and so on; for in itself the will is as wild and impetuous an impulse as is the force appearing in the plunging waterfall; in fact, it is, as we know, ultimately identical therewith.'[66]

Whereas Schopenhauer states in his discussion of metaphysics that everything *is* Will (including the intellect), he implies in passages concerning human psychology that there is a *tension* between a person's will on the one hand and intellect on the other, arriving at rather different conclusions regarding the possibility of autonomous action.

Commentators on Schopenhauer's work are therefore undecided about the amount of freedom that Schopenhauer grants the rational subject.[67] Young, for example, argues that although Schopenhauer may claim that we are not aware of the unconscious grounds or 'secret springs' underlying our actions, this does not mean that human beings can be characterized as completely *irrational*: 'It is...a mistake to insist that only what inhabits (past or present) consciousness can count as the reason for an action. An action can be rational, done, that is, for a reason, where the agent is (and might always remain) unconscious of it.'[68] This 'mistake', Young argues, is based on the Cartesian idea that 'I am my consciousness' and that everything originating in my unconsciousness is therefore neither 'me' nor rational.

Young concludes that Schopenhauer defends instrumental rationality rather than irrationality, because any concept of rationality thinkable at all within a Schopenhauerian framework is instrumental in nature: 'For Schopenhauer…, practical reason has an instrumental, never a constitutive role.'[69] Schopenhauer, in other words, denies that reason can be anything *other* than instrumental since any 'ought' can only be an 'ought' once it triggers something 'in' the self. Young concludes: 'Schopenhauer's examples of unconsciously motivated behaviour are, in fact, examples of highly rational behaviour.'[70]

Although Young makes an interesting point, his interpretation only denies one aspect of the charge that Schopenhauer is an irrationalist. By claiming that Schopenhauer defends rationalism because he tries to show that all actions are based on (in most cases *unknown*) reasons, he does deny that human beings can be rational in the Korsgaardian sense described above, namely as self-constituting and responsible actors. Young's understanding of rationality thereby comes rather close to the idea that even certain non-human animals are rational creatures because some of their actions are based on reasons that they are not aware of. He thereby reduces rationality to the status of a mere tool in the service of the Will and actually ends up affirming Lukács' point that Schopenhauer dismisses the notion of autonomous and critical action instead of defending him against this charge, as he set out to do.

Let us evaluate this same point in light of the above-discussed contrast between, on the one hand, rationally seeking to achieve an end that itself is pre-given by our, to put it in Schopenhauer's terms, unchangeable characters and, on the other hand, rationally determining the ends that we set ourselves. Whereas we, in the first case, are guided by our nature and are unfree as actors, we are, in the second case, free as actors since we ourselves decide what we set out to do and what we want to achieve. Even though Young may be right in claiming that Schopenhauer defends the rational nature of human behaviour according to the first understanding of what it means to be rational, he cannot argue that he does this according to the second understanding of rationality. And this means, again, that he has to agree with a critic like Lukács that Schopenhauer argues that human beings are unfree: they are unable to be guided by rational deliberation since the ends they seek to achieve are always pre-determined by their unchangeable, empirical characters.

Freedom

But Schopenhauer's philosophy does not completely rule out the notion of freedom. Following Kant's dichotomy between the empirical and intelligible characters, he claims that the intelligible character, which he also cryptically defines as one's 'will as thing-in-itself',[71] is free: this character does not know causality, time and space and is not structured by the *principium individuationis*. Schopenhauer concludes:

> Consequently, my exposition does not eliminate freedom. It merely moves it out, namely, out of the area of simple actions, where it demonstrably cannot be found, up to a region which lies higher, but is not so easily accessible to our knowledge. In other words, freedom is transcendental.[72]

But this results in a rather problematic position: Schopenhauer preserves freedom by denying it to human beings. In spite of his above-mentioned problematic suggestion that the intelligible character manifests itself in the world of causality as the empirical character, he now removes it from the realm of action and thought completely and places it in an ungraspable, transcendental beyond that makes it unclear what the shape of the intelligible character is or how it can be part of a person's self at all.[73]

Following these analyses, we therefore have to conclude that Schopenhauer does not grant the faculty of reason anything more than an instrumental function. In *On the Basis of Morality* he even explicitly rejects a Korsgaardian picture of rationality by arguing the following:

> [Rational conduct] by no means implies uprightness and love for one's fellows. On the contrary, a man can go to work very rationally, and thus thoughtfully, deliberately, consistently, systematically, and methodologically, and yet act upon the most selfish, unjust, and even iniquitous maxims.... Reasonable and vicious are quite consistent with each other, in fact, only through their union are great and far-reaching crimes possible.[74]

Even though, as we have seen, Schopenhauer is at places rather unclear about the freedom of the rational subject and claims that the intellect has some control over the Will, his theory as a whole, revolving around a metaphysical and unchangeable essence, eventually forces us to conclude that that the faculty of reason, in his view, can only follow, never lead; it can only assist but never determine. I will briefly return to this issue in Chapter 9 and show that Schopenhauer discusses freedom as well in his analysis of the denial of the Will.

Egotism and the state

Egotism is colossal

In the following, I want to briefly analyse how the three above-discussed forms of rationalism and irrationalism return in Schopenhauer's analysis of egotism. Not only will we see that this phenomenon plays a main role in his moral philosophy, but I will also argue in Chapters 5, 8 and 10 that Schopenhauer's approach to egotistic behaviour returns in Adorno's thought.

Schopenhauer understands egotism as the most prevalent anti-moral incentive in human beings and argues that it follows from a combination of two characteristics of the self. First, egotistic behaviour follows, in his view, from the drive to self-preservation; by a 'craving for existence and well-being'[75] that is 'most intimately connected with [our] most innermost core and essence; in fact, it is really identical with essence'.[76]

Second, he claims that egotism follows from the manner in which we perceive the world-as-representation: as consisting of separate objects and as a world in which every human being, therefore, is separated from every other human being. He observes in this context: 'everyone is given to himself directly, but the rest are given to him only *indirectly* through their representation in his head; and the directness asserts its right. Thus in consequence of subjectivity essential to every consciousness, everyone is himself the whole world'.[77]

With these statements we arrive at Schopenhauer's solution to the problem why we are able to turn a blind eye to the suffering of others. Not only does Schopenhauer affirm that this is often the case, he explains it by referring to *the nature of human beings*. We are 'wired', in his view, to think only about ourselves, to be driven by self-preservation and to perceive the world as permeated by the *principium individuationis*:

> Egoism is colossal; it towers above the world; for if every individual were given the choice between his own destruction and that of the rest of the world, I need not say how the decision would go in the vast majority of cases. Accordingly, everyone makes himself the center of the world, and refers everything to himself. Whatever occurs – for example, the greatest changes in the fate of nations – is first referred to his interests; however small and indirect these may be, they are thought of before anything else.[78]

In this statement the three above-discussed forms of rationalism and irrationalism return. First, we have seen that Schopenhauer is an ontological irrationalist, concluding that the essence of the world and of human beings does not mirror the rational mind. The world is a meaningless whole, he argues, defined by blind Will, and human beings are driven by endless desires and strivings that can never be satisfied completely. One of the strongest of these is the drive to self-preservation, which Schopenhauer understands as the motor behind egotistic behaviour.

Second, our access to the world is irrational as well, he argues. We perceive the world outside of us as permeated with the *principium individuationis,* which is the result of a process – the Understanding – that Schopenhauer defines as irrational in nature and that he also attributes to animals. It is this process that constitutes a world in which we perceive ourselves as separate from others, a world in which egotism blossoms. Furthermore, we experience the world inside of us in an irrational manner too, consisting of drives, desires and strivings that torment us from the day we are born.

However, I have shown that Schopenhauer does argue that we can develop rational insight into these latter experiences, which means that regarding our direct access to the world he can be characterized as an epistemological irrationalist, but that his theory is rationalistic where it concerns our ability to reflect on this access and on the limits of the world-as-representation. This idea returns in his analysis of egotism, which consists of a highly rational analysis of the irrationality of the drive to self-preservation.

Third, I have concluded that Schopenhauer is an irrationalist regarding the ability to rationally control the Will inside of us. Again, this idea returns in his understanding of egotism: we cannot control or suppress the drive to self-preservation, in his view, which forces us to think only about our own well-being.

I have also argued that the first two forms of irrationalism present us with two arguments for Schopenhauer's pessimism. His ontological irrationalism teaches us that the world is meaningless and has no goal. Furthermore, it implies that we are constantly overcome by desires and strivings and that we cannot find permanent satisfaction. His epistemological irrationalism, furthermore, implies that our access to the world is not rational in nature. We are able to rationally analyse the world and the desires we feel inside of ourselves, but this only turns us into powerless onlookers to our enslavement to the Will.

Schopenhauer's focus on the dominant nature of egotism brings us to another argument for pessimism: almost by definition, Schopenhauer claims, human beings do not care about the suffering of others, which makes this world even worse than it already is, in his view. He characterizes this situation by repeating a famous phrase by Plautus, referred to by Thomas Hobbes to characterize the selfish nature of human beings: 'The chief source of the most serious evils affecting man is man himself; homo homini lupus.'[79] Pessimistically, Schopenhauer therefore concludes: 'the world is just a hell and in it human beings are the tortured souls on the one hand, and the devils on the other.'[80]

The state

Even though Schopenhauer's texts do not contain many reflections on politics, his affirmation of irrationality and egotism do result in an understanding of the functions of the state. It is here that I want to return to Lukács' critique: since the above-discussed forms of irrationality – as they are interpreted within Schopenhauer's philosophy – result in the idea that egotism follows from the essence of human beings, his thought eventually culminates in the idea that history does not exist; it is a mere phenomenon that follows from the unchangeable nature of the world and of humanity. Lukács therefore argues that Schopenhauer's thought suggests that every attempt to change the world or the social conditions under which people live is useless and thereby affirms the nature of this world:

> This, then fulfils the task of Schopenhauer's irrationalism: the task of preventing an otherwise dissatisfied sector of the intelligentsia from concretely turning its discontent with the 'established order', that is, the existing social order, against the capitalist system in force at any given time. This irrationalism thereby reaches its central objective – no matter how far Schopenhauer himself was aware of it; that of providing an indirect apologetic of the capitalist social order.[81]

This brings us to Schopenhauer's ideas on politics. Indeed, his understanding of the organization of the state does nothing to overcome or temper egotism or to change the ways in which people believe they are categorically independent of and different from each other. Furthermore, it is not constructed from a point of view that proclaims that the idea that everyone has to compete with everyone else is based on a mere illusion. Again referring to Hobbes, Schopenhauer argues that the prime reason why people organize themselves politically and construct a state is to make sure that no one gets hurt by other people and that every individual can – within limits – develop itself according to its own needs. He furthermore claims that the state should have the right to punish people in order to control their anti-social tendencies and thereby set an example to others.[82]

This means that Schopenhauer's analysis of the functions of the state is based on a cynical affirmation of the observation that the behaviour of most people is driven by egotism and that they cannot change their own characters: only by inciting fear for being punished may the state be able to control its citizens. Furthermore, it is devoid of idealism or hope:

> The State is set up on the correct assumption that pure morality, i.e. the right conduct from moral grounds, is not to be expected; otherwise it itself would be superfluous. Thus the State, aiming at well-being, is by no means directed against egoism, but only against the injurious consequences of egoism arising out of the plurality of egoistic individuals, reciprocally affecting them, and disturbing their well-being.[83]

The state, Schopenhauer goes on, is 'the means by which egoism, endowed with the faculty of reason, seeks to avoid its own evil consequence that turn against itself.'[84] Driven by a desire for its own well-being, in other words, the egoistic individual creates a political situation with other egoistic individuals to ensure its own safety.[85] The organization of a state herewith follows from the ability to rationally reflect on one's situation. Again, however, the faculty of reason here merely follows drives of an egotistic nature and is instrumental in nature.

For a brief moment, however, Schopenhauer's analysis of the state seems to provide us with a glimmer of hope: if the state succeeds in removing 'all kinds of evil', he argues, 'something approaching a Utopia might finally be brought about.'[86] However, he immediately crushes this hope by claiming that when we really think about the nature of the world, we have to conclude that the coming about of this Utopia is impossible. Not only will 'innumerable evils, absolutely essential to life' always keep humanity in suffering, boredom would also immediately reign in this utopian situation. Furthermore, other nations will eventually invade this Utopia and wars will arise, Schopenhauer argues.

And lastly, even if a Utopia were to be constituted, 'the result in the end would be actual over-population of the whole planet, the terrible evil of which only a bold imagination can conjure up in the mind',[87] Schopenhauer argues. In short: Schopenhauer's pessimism forces him to claim that the organization of the state can only be based on egotism and follows from the idea that no happiness can come about through social change:[88] Lukács' judgement therefore seems to be accurate.

It is important to keep in mind, however, that Lukács' interpretation mainly revolves around specific aspects of Schopenhauer's thought. Even though he may not believe in social change, Lukács' claim that Schopenhauer's irrationalism exclusively results in egotism and an 'apologetic of the capitalist social order' overlooks not only Schopenhauer's categorical rejection of suffering and his concern with material needs, but also the fact that his moral philosophy and his aesthetic theory revolve around an overcoming of egotism, to which I return in Chapters 7 and 9. We have already touched upon this aspect in Chapter 3 in the context of Schopenhauer's analysis of compassion. Horkheimer may therefore be rather naive when claiming that Schopenhauer comes close to defending a socialist utopia because he argues that the state would not have to exist if there were no egotism,[89] but we will see in Chapter 8 that Lukács' argument that Schopenhauer merely defends egotism is based on an overly caricaturistic reading of his works as well.[90]

Conclusion

When looking strictly at the three above-discussed ways in which we can read the charge that Schopenhauer is an irrationalist, however, we have to conclude that Lukács is right: Schopenhauer's metaphysical monism makes it impossible for him to claim that human beings have rational control over their destinies; nor can he claim that they are able to change the social and cultural circumstances under which they live. They cannot even rationally change their own behaviour and are destined to live a life characterized by egotism, striving and suffering if we follow Schopenhauer's argument. Freedom, he continually stresses, is found in the passivity of the intelligible character and has nothing to do with the empirical world in which we exist as acting beings.

Furthermore, Lukács is right when he states that for Schopenhauer 'history does not exist': every act, every type of behaviour follows according to him from an unchangeable human essence. The culture in which we live, the concepts through which we think, the social conditions under which we grow up and the historically formed ideas that are prevalent in our times have no influence on who and what we are.

Yukio Mishima's observations, revolving around the ahistorical notion of a split between mind and body, consciousness and flesh, return hereby in Schopenhauer's philosophy with the idea that the rational mind is powerless regarding the overpowering nature of the body as a manifestation of Will. The world itself (which includes our bodies), our access to this world (which takes place through our bodies) and our behaviour (which is defined by our bodies), are ultimately driven by Will in its many forms, and are therefore irrational in nature, Schopenhauer argues.

Even though it is difficult to agree with most of Schopenhauer's above-discussed overly radical arguments, I want to conclude that his observations nevertheless force us to adopt a critical perspective. The grim nature of Schopenhauer's metaphysics makes him pierce through enlightenment ideals like freedom, self-constitution and progress and show us that in most cases people are merely driven by self-preservation or the preservation of their species. Peter Dews quotes a telling statement Schopenhauer made in a conversation towards the end of his life: 'A philosophy in which one does not hear, between the pages, tears, howling and chattering of teeth, and the frightful din of general, reciprocal murder, is no philosophy.'[91] Horkheimer praises this grim and critical aspect of Schopenhauer's thought as follows: 'the doctrine of blind will as an eternal force removes from the world the treacherous gold foil which the old metaphysics had given it. In utter contrast to positivism, it enunciates the negative and preserves it in thought.... No need is ever compensated in any Beyond.'[92]

Schopenhauer's theory urges us to take the (psychoanalytical) claim into account that we do not completely control everything we are; that there is an aspect to our existence that the faculty of reason does not encapsulate entirely. In this context, Christopher Janaway observes that the idea of body and brain as 'manifestations of blind purposiveness' form one of the most important and revolutionary aspects of Schopenhauer's doctrine of the primacy of the will and the unfreedom of the self.[93] Since Schopenhauer, especially in his later works, understands the human body, including the brain, as *manifested Will*, his observations on the difficulties of *really* changing or *knowing* oneself could be translated into the idea that we *are* our bodies, to the idea that our behaviour, thoughts, ideas and plans are dependent on rather ungraspable bodily processes.[94]

As I have argued in Chapters 2 and 3, we again see that the naturalistic tendencies of Schopenhauer's philosophy introduce an interesting dimension to his ideas. Even though we may not agree with his conclusions about the completely determined nature of human behaviour, I do think that we should value his attempt to confront Kant's philosophy with observations regarding our corporeal nature.[95] Even though Schopenhauer's conclusions might be too extreme, in other words, his philosophy forces us to take the idea into account that we are dependent on processes over which we do not have complete rational control.

5
The Whole Is the Wrong

Introduction

Samuel Beckett's play *Endgame* consists of one act and has four characters: Hamm, who is blind and cannot stand, Clov, Hamm's servant who cannot sit, and Hamm's parents, Nagg and Nell, who both have no legs and live in dustbins. These four characters are not able to really communicate with each other; they either utter absurdist phrases or vaguely reflect on their situation without arriving at definitive conclusions. The play is devoid of human warmth and takes place in a house that is surrounded by a world that is characterized as 'corpsed'.[1]

In his lectures on *Metaphysics*, Adorno states that the dramas of Beckett are the 'only truly relevant metaphysical productions since the war'.[2] Like no other modern works of art, he argues, they represent the horrors of Auschwitz, to which he frequently refers when evaluating the modern world, the course of history, and the faculty of reason that human beings developed to grasp their environment. Adorno especially praises Beckett's emphasis on corporeality and pain, as well as his ability to describe the state of existence to which people were reduced in the concentration camps, consisting of a physical suffering that 'already places the living man among the corpses by reducing him to his body'.[3]

But the play's four characters' inability to communicate also reflects philosophy's inability to really say something meaningful about the barbarity of the death camps, Adorno states. In a sense, he argues, the human catastrophe that he refers to with the word 'Auschwitz', as well as the social and historical conditions that resulted in the barbarity of Nazi Germany, overshadow and corrode the thinking and feeling subject to such an extent that it is as damaged and unfree – both in a physical and conceptual sense – as the characters in *Endgame*.

With this transformation from a metaphysical to a social 'wrong whole' we arrive at one of the main differences between Schopenhauer and Adorno, which was emphasized in the Introduction to this book. Whereas one can find observations on the nature of civilization in Schopenhauer's philosophy – Adorno even groups Schopenhauer with Hegel among those who speak 'cuttingly of the horrors of history'[4] – these observations do not play an important role in his understanding of the self. Strongly influenced by Marx, Hegel and Weber's ideas, Adorno argues, *pace* Schopenhauer, that the thinking and experiencing subject is always formed in a historical, social and linguistic context and cannot be understood outside of it.[5]

However, in this chapter I aim to show that certain tendencies and ideas that can be found in Schopenhauer's thought do return in Adorno's philosophy. In the latter's lectures on *Negative Dialectics*, we find the following passage on Hegel: 'Hegel should be defended against the old slur on "the strait-jacket of dialectics". It is the strait-jacket of the world.'[6] In *At the Mind's Limits*, to which I return in Chapter 6, a similar idea is reflected by Jean Améry, who describes the experience of being imprisoned in a concentration camp as follows:

> The power structure of the SS state towered up before the prisoner monstrously and indomitably, a reality that could not be escaped and that therefore finally seemed reasonable. No matter what his thinking may have been on the outside, in this sense here he became a Hegelian: in the metallic brilliance of its totality the SS state appeared as a state in which the idea was becoming reality.[7]

I will argue that it is this idea of 'being imprisoned' *within* a way of thinking, within the 'strait-jacket of the world', within 'that objective *machine infernale* from which consciousness ... would like to escape'[8] – a historical condition that Hegel's theory on history ironically reflects, in Adorno's view – that forms a returning theme in Adorno's understanding of the subject and that makes his bleak observations on the weak and almost diminished self into a historicized version of Schopenhauer's pessimistic observations on the tragic aspects of human existence.

In order to develop this argument, this chapter contains an overview of the historical observations on which Adorno's grim diagnosis of modernity rests. Following the analysis of Schopenhauer's understanding of rationality, developed in Chapter 4, I will mainly focus on Adorno's discussions of the rise of the rational self and the dominance of self-preservation, and show how and where they are similar to several of Schopenhauer's observations.

It should be kept in mind that the discussion in this chapter will be rather superficial: its scope does not allow me to discuss all aspects of Adorno's critique of modernity in depth. It mainly serves as a way to shed a first light on the similarities and differences between Schopenhauer and Adorno's ideas on the self and forms a stepping stone towards more detailed analyses of the latter's philosophy in Chapters 6, 8 and 10.

The bear's teeth

In order to understand Adorno's notion of the self, we have to look at *Dialectic of Enlightenment*, which he wrote with Horkheimer while in exile from Germany in the United States during the last years of the war. In this book, which made Habermas group Adorno and Horkheimer with Nietzsche and De Sade among 'the black writers of the bourgeoisie',[9] the authors analyse the state of modern, enlightened culture and develop a highly critical notion of the modern self in which several aspects of Schopenhauer's philosophy return.

One of these Schopenhauerian tendencies is the observation that Adorno does not claim that things used to be better in a pre-modern age, before the enlightenment. He dismisses any belief in a pre-18th century healthy culture as a romantic and ideological illusion, a 'cliché of the Golden Age'[10] created by the same culture he criticizes.[11] There has never been a 'better' or 'healthier' society, Adorno observes: atrocities and genocide have always been committed, and in that sense the human catastrophes that took place during Adorno's lifetime do not form an exception, merely a radical intensification of already existing tendencies and mechanisms. He states dramatically: 'no universal history leads from savagery to humanitarianism, but there is one leading from the slingshot to the megaton bomb.'[12] In a passage on Marx' analysis of natural history, furthermore, he claims in a rather Schopenhauerian mood: 'human history, the history of the progressing mastery of nature, continues the unconscious history of nature, of devouring and being devoured.'[13]

This does not mean, however, that human beings have been and will always be the same. The 'modern self' that Adorno criticizes consists of a historically formed pathologization of a specific kind of rationality, which implies that the subject may relate differently to itself and its environment under different social conditions. I return to these ideas below.

Adorno analyses the mechanisms that constitute the modern self in the first excursus in *Dialectic of Enlightenment* by developing a symbolic representation of the rise of a specific type of consciousness. He links this type of consciousness to Odysseus, the hero of Homer's *Odyssey*, who is understood by Adorno as the prototype of a civilized and enlightened subject. The essence of Adorno's interpretation is symbolized by the trick Odysseus develops to be able to enjoy the deadly song of the Sirens and survive the experience: he puts wax in the ears of his rowers and lets them tie him to the mast of his ship. When they pass the Sirens, Odysseus screams and commands his rowers to untie him and let him disappear into the pleasurable but deadly arms of the Sirens, but his rowers do not hear anything. They quietly row further until they are out of the reach of the deadly creatures.

Odysseus has hereby used his ability to rationally reflect on his situation to control the forces of pleasure and death that surround him. His survey over the world, his capacity to schematize nature *and* his own desires has enabled him to survive the non-survivable. Odysseus, in Adorno's view, is the first man who actually breaks the spell of nature and to withdraw himself from its seemingly necessary cycle. He therefore forms the embodiment of enlightenment-thinking: 'Technically enlightened, Odysseus acknowledges the archaic supremacy of the song by having himself bound.... The epic does not say what happens to the singers once the ship has passed. But in a tragedy this would have been their last hour'.[14] By mastering natural, mythical and cyclical forces, Odysseus has destroyed their power.

Like Schopenhauer, Adorno here argues that the faculty of reason originates in the drive to self-preservation; being rational allows one to master one's environment and one's instincts and control them in the service of one's survival, he suggests. The naturalistic and, again, Schopenhauerian tendencies of this claim should not be underestimated. In 'On the Critique of the Philosophy of History', in the last section of *Dialectic of Enlightenment*, for example, we find the following observation on rationality:

> The human species is not, as has been asserted, a freak event in natural history, an incidental and abnormal formation produced by hypertrophy of the cerebral organ.... The cerebral organ, human intelligence, is firmly established enough to constitute a regular epoch of the earth's history. In this epoch, the human species, including its machines, chemicals, and organizational powers – for why should they not be seen as a part of it as teeth are a part of the bear, since they serve the same purpose and merely function better? – is the last word in adaptation. Humans have not only overtaken their immediate

> predecessors but have eradicated them more thoroughly than almost any other recent species, not excluding the carnivorous saurians.[15]

In the last paragraph of the 'Notes and Sketches' in the same book, the authors furthermore develop the following metaphor:

> The emblem of intelligence is the feeler of the snail.... Meeting an obstacle, the feeler is immediately withdrawn into the protection of the body, it becomes one with the whole until it timidly ventures forth again as an autonomous agent. If the danger is still present, it disappears once more, and the intervals between the attempts grow longer. Mental life in its earliest stages is infinitely delicate. The snail's sense is dependent on a muscle and muscles grow slack if their scope for movement is impaired. The body is crippled by physical injury, the mind by fear. In their origin both effects are inseparable. The highest animals have themselves to thank for their greater freedom; their existence is evidence that feelers were once stretched out in new directions and not repulsed. Each of their species is a monument to countless others whose attempts to develop were blocked at the outset; which gave way to fright if only a single feeler stirred in the path of their evolution.[16]

The observation that intelligence has developed like the teeth of a bear or like the feeler of a snail, devouring its prey or instinctively stretching out into a darkness of which it is afraid but which it nevertheless aims to grasp, could have been developed by Schopenhauer. In fact, it bears resemblance to a passage in *On the Will in Nature*, where Schopenhauer argues, with reference to Lamarck, that the different bodily functions and abilities developed by different species – including the intellect – are driven by Will: 'the snail was originally, like other *mollusca,* without feelers; but out of the desire to feel the objects lying before it, these gradually arose'.[17]

Instrumental reason

Self-constitution as self-sacrifice

Although originating in a natural drive, although growing out of the instinctual body like the feeler out of the snail, Adorno argues that the faculty of reason eventually elevated itself out of nature. This brings us to his diagnosis of the pathological character of reason and of the modern, rational self. Through this elevation, Adorno argues, reason turns back upon the entity out of which it rose, permeating and encapsulating it: Odysseus constitutes his autonomy and individuality by developing a *controlling* attitude towards internal and external nature and in that same moment *distances* himself from both himself and the world. He has to tie *himself* to the mast of his ship in order to survive. Adorno herewith argues that 'self-assertion, as in the entire epic, as in all civilization, is self-repudiation':[18]

> The human being's mastery of itself, on which the self is founded, practically always involves the annihilation of the subject in whose service that mastery is maintained, because the substance which is mastered, suppressed, and disintegrated by self-preservation is nothing other than the living entity, of which the achievements of self-preservation can only be defined as functions – in other words, self-preservation destroys the very thing which is to be preserved.[19]

Odysseus' instinctual need to protect himself forces him to control and to aggressively dominate everything that may form a threat to his self. He does this by separating himself from all that ties him to nature, from everything that he cannot rationally control – thereby eventually distorting his *own* natural dimension as well, violently repressing any need, desire, feeling or emotion that pulls him back into the unexpectedness of nature.

Adorno's claim that the origins of rationality lie in the drive to self-preservation, furthermore, implies that the subject that is the result of this process is not defined by an *opposition* between nature and reason but an *entwinement* of self-preservation and rationality. This, in turn, constitutes *instrumental rationality*, which in the service of self-preservation celebrates an irrational and blind suppression of everything that can harm or endanger the ego: 'pure reason became unreason, a procedure as immune to errors as it was devoid of content.'[20] The faculty of reason, in this reading, fuelled by the drive to self-preservation, eventually turns into its opposite.

Whereas Schopenhauer strikingly anticipated the insights of psychoanalysis, Adorno here almost literally repeats Freud's observations in *Civilization and its Discontents* on the rise of a super-ego that turns against the ego. In Freud's words: 'Civilization ... obtains mastery over the individual's dangerous desire for aggression by weakening and disarming it and by setting up an agency within him to watch over it, like a garrison in a conquered city.'[21]

Following Freud, Adorno intrinsically connects the formation of the civilization he analyses and eventually criticizes to the process of rational self-constitution, implying that this civilization is inherently rooted in violence. Since, as briefly mentioned above, he approaches rationality, as well as the ways in which we reflect on ourselves and others in a rather Hegelian manner as permeated with social categories, the above-described elevation out of nature by way of rational self-control is understood by him as a social process, as the incorporation of social norms and values that repress everything *within this same self* that does not conform to these norms or is considered to be a threat – I return below to the details of his analysis of this social dimension.

Bodily alienation

Within the context of this book, it is important to notice that Adorno explicitly refers to a violent repression of the *body*: Odysseus has to tie his body to the mast of his ship. Whereas this claim contains a Marxist critical analysis of the division of labour – Odysseus instrumentalizes his rowers by letting them perform physical work for him and remaining passive himself (I return to Marx below) – Adorno also implies that civilized and enlightened men distort or even lose a certain relationship with their bodies by forming a self. This claim is made even more explicitly in a paragraph on the 'Interest in the body' in *Dialectic of Enlightenment*, in which Adorno positions his analysis of self-constitution in a social context: 'Beneath the known history of Europe there runs a subterranean one. It consists of the fate of the human instincts and passions repressed and distorted by civilization'[22] and: 'love-hate for the body colors the whole of modern culture. The body is scorned and rejected as something inferior, enslaved, and at the same time as forbidden, reified, estranged.'[23]

Civilization is understood as creating a gap, a *chorismos* between ego and body through a violent repression *of* this body. As Adorno writes in *Negative Dialectics*: 'The separation of the sensual and intellectual realms... is a social product; by the *chorismos,* sensuality is designated as a victim of the intellect.'[24] In his article on Adorno and Freud, Joel Whitebook insightfully shows how Adorno herewith pits 'the claims of the *material* body against the (ideological) illusions of theoretical and moral idealism'.[25] This theme will return in Chapter 8.

This means that Odysseus *preserves himself by rejecting himself,* he survives by violently 'subsuming, classifying, subordinating' and 'cutting short'[26] his natural dimension. Again, the naturalistic tendencies within this analysis should not be underestimated. In this context, we find the following helpful passage in Horkheimer's *Eclipse of Reason*:

> If one were to speak of a disease affecting reason, this disease should be understood not as having stricken reason at some historical moment, but as being inseparable from the nature of reason in civilization as we have known it so far. The disease of reason is that reason was born from man's urge to dominate nature, and the 'recovery' depends on insight into the nature of the original disease, not on a cure of the latest symptoms.[27]

Adorno's observations on the pervasive and overpowering nature of the rational subject, fuelled by a violent and pathological drive to control and dominate everything that is 'other', do not only result in the claim that this subject itself is corroded by its own pathological need to control. He also argues that the world this subject lives in is fundamentally corrupted, manipulated and instrumentalized:

> This kind of rationality exists only in so far as it can subjugate something different from and alien to itself. We can put it even more strongly: it can exist only by identifying everything that is caught up in its machinery, by levelling it and by defining it in its alterity as something that resists it and, we may even go so far as to say, something that is hostile to it.[28]

Any access to the world and to one's self is blocked and distorted by this kind of rationality, since it 'spins a web around its objects that leaves fewer and fewer gaps for everything that is not itself'.[29]

Commodification and second nature

The totalizing negativity and the all-engulfing pessimism with which Adorno approaches the resulting world equals the bleakness of Schopenhauer's observations. But in order to compare Adorno's thoughts on corporeality and rationality with those of Schopenhauer, we first have to look more precisely at the specific levels and implications of the former's critique of instrumental reason.

This brings us to the way in which Adorno translates his above-discussed ideas on the birth of the self into a critical analysis of social conditions in modernity. He mainly does this within a framework inspired by Marx's understanding of commodification, developed in the first volume of *Capital*.[30]

In the paragraph 'The fetishism of the commodity and its secret', Marx analyses the development of an economic system in which goods can be exchanged. Since such a system makes it possible for people to become less dependent on that which they produce themselves and increases their chances of survival, the development of such an economic system is steered by the drive to self-preservation, like Odysseus' elevation out of nature in Adorno's interpretation.

In order to create this economic system, the use-value of a product has to be replaced by exchange-value, Marx argues. Whereas the first concept refers to the value a product has for a particular person in a particular situation, the second kind of value determines what other products it can be traded for. This latter value was originally based on the average time needed to produce a product, Marx claims.[31] Determining the exchange-value of products in this way makes it possible, in other words, to compare products with each other and to trade them within a market-system.

This emphasis on shared value and on average production time, Marx observes, robs products of their individual and particular qualities and transforms them into what he calls 'commodities'. As commodities, products are no longer valued by their particular qualities and the individual skills needed to produce them, but are approached from a general point of view and provided with a value that is based on a non-existing standard that is only created to compare them. Commodities hereby gain a 'mystical character',[32] of which Marx writes that it has 'absolutely no connection with the physical nature of the commodity and the material relations arising out of it'.[33]

But since capitalist societies revolve around profit and since profit is made by way of a market-system based on exchange, Marx argues that within this society more and more products become standardized and commodified, which eventually results in the 'finished form of the world of commodities – the money form.'[34] Money became the universal way of comparing and trading goods, he claims, because it makes it possible to not only measure the value of products in a standardized manner, but also the value of time, labour and, eventually, people.

This process of commodification and standardization, driven by the ever-growing need to produce surplus-value, eventually results in the phenomenon of alienation, Marx famously observes. Workers are disconnected from the products of their work: they are placed on assembly lines, for example, made part of only a small aspect of the production process.

Furthermore, people become alienated from each other and the world in which they live: once more and more spheres of life are permeated with a standardizing system according to which everything and everyone can be valued in terms of money, these spheres lose their particular and individual nature. And since money makes it possible to measure the value of labour power, generalizing the individual work that particular people do for the people who own of the means of production, this eventually makes relations between people 'appear as relations between material objects'[35] and reduces them to 'objects of utility', Marx claims.[36]

The process of commodification hereby transforms people, like products, into mere functions in an equation that has to result in profit, robbing them of their individuality and making them into mere parts of a machine. Furthermore, Marx argues, commodification enhances domination, not only of the workers (who are reduced to functions in an equation), but also of nature and of natural resources, which are perceived from a standardized and efficiency-focused standpoint and robbed of their intrinsic value and their individual and particular nature.

For Adorno, a crucial aspect of Marx's analysis consists of the idea that the process of commodification eventually appears as a 'natural law'. Marx writes:

> What initially concerns producers in practice when they make an exchange is how much of some other product they get for their own; in what proportions can the products be exchanged? As soon as these proportions have attained a certain customary ability, they appear to result from the nature of the products.[37]

This idea was further developed by Georg Lukács in *History and Class Consciousness*, which had an important influence on Adorno's philosophy. Lukács describes Marx's analysis as follows, developing the concept of 'second nature':

> [M]en are constantly smashing, replacing, and leaving behind the 'natural,' irrational, and actually existing bonds, while, on the other hand, they erect around themselves in the reality that they have created and 'made,' a kind of second nature which evolves with exactly the same inexorable necessity as was the case earlier with irrational forces of nature.[38]

This process, which makes the 'mysterious' and, according to Marx, completely superficial commodity character of a product appear as its true nature, has dramatic consequences. Now, Lukács observes: 'the powers that are beyond man's control assume quite a different character', which appears 'as the ineluctable consequence of known, knowable, rational systems of laws, as a necessity which cannot ultimately and wholly be grasped'.[39] The process of commodification, in other words, not only permeates more and more aspects of society – dominating people, nature and work – but also appears as *rational*, necessary and unchangeable, as the way things are and will always be, and thereby controls the manner in which people experience themselves and their environment.

The modern self

Self-preservation and domination

Developing his critique of modernity, Adorno entwines Marx's notion of commodification with the above-discussed analysis of instrumental rationality, which he constructs in his interpretation of the *Odyssey*. Both the process of commodification and the constitution of the modern self go hand in hand with generalization and standardization, he argues. Most importantly, both revolve around a dominating attitude towards people and nature, robbing the particular of its individual nature, subsuming it under broad categories and only approaching it by relating it to the needs of the dominating self. Furthermore, both are driven by a drive to self-preservation that slowly turns into a dominating force.

The scope of this chapter does not allow me to discuss the subtleties and complexities of Marx's philosophy or of Adorno's reading of Marx. However, the above-developed brief (and of course incomplete) sketch of Marx's analysis of commodification and of Lukács' emphasis on the transformation from first to second nature, makes it possible to show that Adorno argues that the process of commodification has gained such an autonomous and independent character that it not only controls modern societies to a large extent, but its appearance as necessity makes it almost impossible to pierce through its veil and unmask its illusory nature. It has gained the ability to determine the needs people have and the ends they set themselves and thereby diminishes their freedom, even when they themselves may think that they are free: 'The law of value comes into play over the heads of formally free individuals. They are unfree, according to Marx's insight, as the involuntary executors of that law.'[40] As Adorno puts this in one of his lectures: 'in that second nature, in our universal state of dependency, there is no freedom.'[41]

Whereas Marx famously argued that the internal contradictions of the capitalist system would eventually result in its collapse, and whereas Lukács claimed that the methodology developed by Marx allows us to rationally pierce through the false nature of capitalist societies and constitute social action, Adorno arrives at a more pessimistic conclusion and observes that the overpowering nature of this system of commodification has actually resulted in its preservation. It has done this by distributing the profit that the system as a whole made in a better way than Marx predicted, thereby increasing the quality of life of most people within capitalist societies. But most of all, it has done this by permeating through all spheres of society to such an extent that the 'mystical character' of commodities appears as completely true and 'objective', which has resulted in the above-mentioned 'Hegelian strait-jacket'. Even though people are reduced to mere cogs in a social machine, and even though relations between people are mediated by efficiency and an emphasis on profit, this means that they believe themselves to be free, Adorno observes. The commodification of society hereby buries both the unfreedom that characterizes this society and the power relations and domination on which it is based, and hides them behind an illusory veil.

Four aspects of modernity

In order to make these rather totalizing and abstract claims more concrete, I want to discuss four spheres of modern life within which Adorno discerns the mechanisms of commodification and standardization. The first is philosophy and, more specifically, what Adorno calls 'identity-thinking'.[42] Since philosophy is conceptual in nature, Adorno argues, it always partly fails to grasp its 'other', fails to grasp the particularity and individuality of that which it refers to. As he puts this in *Negative Dialectics*: 'An object can be conceived only by a subject but always remains something other than the subject.'[43] Conceptual thought, in other words, is never entirely able to do justice to the *non-identity* of the object.

This is a general aspect of conceptuality, Adorno argues, but in modernity the idea has been uncritically embraced that the subject can completely grasp the object. Herewith, he mainly refers to the kind of thinking that he associates with enlightenment thought, scientific progress and positivism. Within these traditions, Adorno observes, philosophy is understood as completely mirroring reality. He argues that when it is guided by this idea, philosophy acquires the rather aggressive tendency to make everything equal to itself, not unlike exchange-value eradicates the particular and individual characteristics of a specific product; and not unlike the way in which Odysseus developed the ability to master and dominate his environment by rationally reflecting on it and schematizing it.

This observation forms the basis of Adorno's quite aggressive attack on existential phenomenology in *The Jargon of Authenticity*, in which he criticizes mainly Heidegger for fetishizing concepts like 'Being' and 'Authenticity' by avoiding their conceptual nature.[44] But Adorno also criticizes Hegel for developing a dialectical system that eventually results in the overcoming of dialectical tensions and in the usurpation of the non-identical by the identical: Hegel's dialectics, he argues, seeks 'to eliminate the moment that cannot be fully absorbed.'[45] As briefly mentioned above, Adorno indeed often refers to Hegel's system as reflecting the all-including wrongness of the social whole, leaving no room for the particular.

Second, Adorno argues that the instrumental rationality he criticizes results in a pathological celebration of technology, which was originally 'the epitome of the means of self-preservation of the human species',[46] but gradually became an end instead of a means, instrumentalizing the environment, human beings and animals, and replacing the intrinsic good of their well-being and flourishing with a celebration of technological progress. Marx's analysis of commodification returns here, according to which the means used to produce products, exchange them and better the quality of life eventually turned into domination, exploitation and alienation. The irrationality of this technology is symbolized by the mass-destruction made possible by the atom bomb to which Adorno refers frequently, implying that, so far, violence and hostility have gone hand in hand with Western progress.[47]

Third, Adorno describes the industry of death that he generally refers to with the word 'Auschwitz'. In his view, the instrumental rationality that revolves around an irrational and blind celebration of self-preservation and a violent approach toward that which is 'other', transformed into the idea of being part of one's people or of one's country's preservation and into feelings of hatred towards everything and everyone depicted as 'different'. It thereby eventually resulted in an irrational and blind pursuit of aggressiveness and industrialized torture on a rational and *planned* level.[48]

Fourth, Adorno refers to what he and Horkheimer in *Dialectic of Enlightenment* call the 'culture industry': a consumption culture consisting of a 'unified system'[49] that manipulates people's needs, thoughts and experiences by pushing them into a pre-fabricated and false image force-fed to the masses through television, radio and movies.

As an example relevant for this chapter, we could think of the experience of sexual pleasure. An important part of Adorno's critique of this 'culture industry' consists of the idea that we are bombarded with sexual imagery, with images of beautiful bodies as well as with pornographic photos and films – 'cellophane-wrapped examples of sex'[50] – that permeate and eventually *distort* the ways in which we experience our bodies, the bodies of others, and the sexual impulses and desires of ourselves and others.[51]

In his 1963 'Sexual Taboos and Law Today', Adorno even argues that it is impossible to speak of sexuality anymore, criticizing the idea of sexual liberation as a 'mere illusion',[52] blind to what he calls the 'desexualization of sexuality'.[53] Pleasure has been standardized and hence eradicated by a 'sex industry' that on the one hand seeks to control and forbid any indecency or 'perversity', and on the other perpetuates a commercialized and false image of what pleasure can be:

> Pleasure that is either kept cornered or accepted with smiling complaisance is no longer pleasure at all; psychoanalysts would be able to demonstrate without difficulty that in the entire sex industry – monopolistically controlled and standardized as it is, with its ready-made appliqués of film stars – fore-pleasure and pleasure-substitutes have surpassed pleasure itself. The neutralization of sex, which has been traced in the disappearance of grand passion, blanches sex even where it is believed to be unabashedly satisfied.[54]

Adorno furthermore argues that the more this 'industry' distorts our ideas about sex and the more violently our sexuality is thereby ignored or repressed, the more aggressive it becomes, 'hidden' under the surface. These repressed libidinal forces are therefore 'ready to be exploited by manipulative powers', which means that no happiness can be found in sexual pleasure, in his view.[55] To a certain extent, Schopenhauer's negative descriptions of endless bodily feelings and needs herewith find their social counterpart in Adorno's ideas about needs and desires that are continually manufactured by the culture industry in such a way that they cannot really be satisfied or result in profound happiness or pleasure.

These four aspects of Adorno's critique of enlightenment-thinking do not refer to completely separate phenomena: the violence that the concept in its universality does to the individual object, Adorno suggests, reflects the violence done to individual human beings in the death camps and to particular and individual experiences – like those of love or sexual pleasure – in the culture industry. Adorno writes in

Negative Dialectics that 'in the concentration camps it was no longer an individual who died, but a specimen.'[56] He therefore understands the politics of Nazi Germany as a radicalization of the process of commodification: under the conditions shaped by these political ideas, individuals are subsumed under general concepts, robbed of their particularity and intrinsic value, treated as mere cogs in a machine and made into 'objects of utility'[57] and eventually into dispensable objects, like the prisoner in Kafka's *In the Penal Colony*.

Coldness and the *principium individuationis*

A reflection of the 'corpsed' whole that is the result of these four aspects of instrumental rationality is found in Adorno's extremely personal observations in *Minima Moralia: Reflections from Damaged Life*, a collection of aphorisms that was released in 1951 and that he dedicated to Max Horkheimer. Adorno characterizes these aphorisms, the title of which is an inversion of Aristotle's *Magna Moralia*, as a 'melancholy science'[58] (as opposed to Nietzsche's *The Gay science*[59]). He writes that it revolves around the classic notion of ethics – 'the teaching of the good life'[60] – and that it attempts to answer the following question: What kind of life can be lived in a whole that is wrong? As Müller-Doohm observes in his biography of Adorno, *Minima Moralia* hereby follows French moralists like La Rochefoucauld, but also Schopenhauer's *Aphorismen zur Lebensweisheit* and Nietzsche's *Menschliches, Allzumenschliches*.[61]

In *Minima Moralia*, Adorno describes a world in which the subject is reduced to a mere shadow, deemed to reflect on its own loss of autonomy, on its own unfreedom, with no means to change this situation. It has lost grasp on itself and its environment. Every possible experience, every communicative action has been usurped and standardized by the culture industry, robbed of its meaning and embedded in a world that is wrong.

One of the main characteristics of this world is a corrosion of meaningful and compassionate relationships between people, for which Adorno frequently uses the term 'coldness'. In *Negative Dialectics*, he describes coldness as 'the basic principle of bourgeois subjectivity, without which there could have been no Auschwitz'.[62] In 'Education After Auschwitz', furthermore, we find the following passage: 'The silence under the terror was only its consequence. The coldness of the societal monad, the isolated competitor, was the precondition, as indifference to the fate of others, for the fact that only very few people reacted. The torturers know this, and they put it to the test ever anew'.[63] Adorno directly links this attitude of coldness to the inescapable and all-permeating nature of the 'wrong whole': 'the very movement of withdrawal bears features of what it negates. It is forced to develop a coldness indistinguishable from that of the bourgeois'.[64]

Warm relationships between people are replaced, according to Adorno's analysis, by a cold and instrumentalizing attitude that reduces subjects to disconnected, individuated atoms. Paradoxically, people thereby become more individuated and disconnected from each other, whereas the process through which this happens is deeply social in nature. Adorno herewith follows Marx, who argues, as we have seen above, that the process of commodification makes relations between people appear as relations between things, which reduces them to 'objects of utility' that only appear as valuable when they fit in a whole mediated by efficiency, profit and money.

Frequently, Adorno refers to Schopenhauer's analysis of the *principium individuationis* to illustrate this observation. In Chapters 2, 3 and 4 we have seen that, for Schopenhauer, the world we perceive necessarily consists of separate and distinct objects. Furthermore, he argues that this world-as-representation is an illusion and refers to it as the 'veil of Maya', which covers a world of 'oneness' that is the real essence of the universe. Adorno transforms these ideas into a historical analysis of the society and culture he criticizes:

> Society determines the individuals to be what they are, even by their immanent genesis. Their freedom or unfreedom is not primary, as it would seem under the veil of the *principium individuationis*. For the ego, as Schopenhauer explained by the myth of Maya's veil, makes even the insight into its dependence difficult to gain for the subjective consciousness. The principle of individualization, the law of particularity to which the universal reason in the individuals is tied, tends to insulate them from the encompassing contexts, and thereby strengthens their flattering confidence in the subject's autarky.[65]

The idea that every individual is separated from every other individual, that every being is self-sufficient and therefore not dependent on other beings or on society, is an illusion that makes people blind to the observation that they are deeply historical and social creatures, Adorno observes.

This brings us to one of the main similarities between Schopenhauer and Adorno. According to Schopenhauer's philosophy the subject is unfree since it is essentially part of a larger whole ('Will'), even though it perceives the world as consisting of distinct phenomena. According to Adorno's philosophy, the subject is unfree since it is part of a larger whole as well (a wrong society), even though it perceives itself as a self-sufficient creature. It may think that it is free and determines its own ends, but in reality, Adorno argues, this is not the case since the way it thinks about itself and experiences its place in the world is defined by social norms and standards. In fact, his analysis of the *Odyssey* suggests that its existence as a self is based on the incorporation of social norms that dominate its nature: 'Even where men are most likely to feel free from society, in the strength of their ego, they are society's agents at the same time. The ego principle is implanted in them by society, and society rewards that principle although it curbs it.'[66]

Schopenhauer's observation that 'egoism towers above the world'[67] echoes through this analysis as well. Adorno repeats this idea in *Negative Dialectics* and gives it a historical twist: 'Temporarily, the individual looms above the blind social context, but in his windowless isolation he only helps so much more to reproduce that context.'[68]

Conclusion

The above-discussed analysis of Adorno's critique of modernity is brief and rather sketchy. I have only been able to scratch the surface of his reading of Marx and his understanding of instrumental rationality, and have mainly tried to argue that whereas Schopenhauer characterizes the subject as powerless because it originates in 'Will', Adorno diagnoses the modern subject with a powerlessness caused by its imprisonment in a pathological rationality that closes this subject off from the world, itself and other people, which results in a commodified social whole defined by coldness and the *principium individuationis*. In his lectures on *History and Freedom*, the dichotomy between 'inside' and 'outside', between 'inner' and 'outer', indeed returns several times as having originated with this distorting wall of rationality, a wall that the enlightened subject initially erected to protect itself against the outside world but that eventually became a mere prison when it paradoxically turned against itself and constructed social and economic mechanisms that standardized and eradicated particularity.[69]

Adorno hereby historicizes Schopenhauer's claim that the self is ultimately unknowable because it is constituted by a transcending and ungraspable striving, and transforms it into a Marxist critique:

> Precisely as an absolute, the individual is a mere reflection of property relations. In him the fictitious claim is made that what is biologically

> one must logically precede the social whole, from which it is only isolated by force, and its contingency is held up as a standard of truth. Not only is the self entwined in society; it owes society its existence in the most literal sense.[70]

Adorno adds: 'the real self has already become in the world what Schopenhauer recognized it to be in introspection, a phantom.'[71]

At several places, Adorno therefore criticizes the existentialist idea of an autonomous and free subject that is able to control and resist its environment. Herewith, we return to Beckett's *Endgame*, discussed in the introduction to this chapter. In his essay on the playwright, Adorno pierces with a Schopenhauerian sharpness through Sartre's, in his view, naïve understanding of individuality: 'Sartre even affirmed the freedom of the victims of the concentration camps to inwardly accept or reject the tortures inflicted upon them. *Endgame* destroys such illusions. The individual himself is revealed to be a historical category.'[72] Hereby, the metaphysical character of Schopenhauer's inversion of Leibniz's dictum into the claim that this is the worst of all possible worlds finds its historical counterpart in Adorno's inversion of Hegel's famous dictum into 'the whole is the wrong'.[73]

6
The Twitching of the Hand

Introduction

Adorno observes in *Negative Dialectics*: 'For thought there is really no other possibility, no other opportunity, than to do what the miner's adage forbids: to work one's way through the darkness without a lamp.'[1] The overpowering bleakness of the social, political and cultural context he analyses makes it difficult, almost impossible, he observes, to find an escape from the status quo, to find the freedom to act or even to think in a world that he characterizes as a 'strait-jacket',[2] and in a culture in which 'there is not even the possibility of something outside it becoming visible, something that is not caught up in the general inclusiveness'.[3]

It is for this reason that Lukács placed Adorno in the 'Grand Hotel Abyss', together with Schopenhauer, as discussed in the Introduction to this book. Both Schopenhauer and Adorno, Lukács argues, affirm the overpowering nature of the whole in which the subject finds itself and thereby undermine the idea that we are able, as rational and autonomous creatures, to grasp our environment and attempt to change it for the better. This results in a fatalistic and passive acceptance of the horrors of the world that leaves no room for the actual possibility of change, to set oneself in motion and attempt to revise the structures that dominate the world, Lukács claims.

A similar point was made by Jürgen Habermas, who famously stated that Horkheimer and Adorno 'surrendered themselves to an uninhibited scepticism regarding reason, instead of weighing the grounds that cast doubt on this scepticism itself'.[4] In Habermas' view, this 'really problematic move' results in an almost universal condemnation of the capacities of reason and a dismissal of its potential for the constitution of autonomy.[5] The almost totalizingly negative tendencies of Adorno's philosophy hereby seem to push him into the same camp as Schopenhauer's ahistorical formulation of the enslavement of reason by Will: according to both, the subject seems to be too unfree to be able to influence itself or the conditions under which it lives.

This is ironic, since Adorno explicitly tried to distance himself from Schopenhauer's ahistorical essentialism. In his lectures on *History and Freedom*, for example, he follows Lukács and criticizes the 'totalising view' of Schopenhauer's pessimism for destroying the possibility that things could be different and for not believing in the idea of rational emancipation. Schopenhauer's philosophy, Adorno writes, 'tends to leap to the assistance of individual evil in the world. It does so by arguing that attempts to change the world as a whole are doomed'.[6]

In the following, I want to look at the manner in which Adorno tries to distinguish the dark nature of his own philosophy from Schopenhauer's pessimistic conclusions. Following Lukács' and Habermas' critiques, I will do this by analysing Adorno's understanding of rationality and by discussing which aspects of the faculty of reason he praises. This discussion will bring us to Adorno's references to the body as well, especially to his ideas on the connection between reason and corporeality. Since Adorno's analysis of rationality, like Schopenhauer's, is mainly based on a reading of Kant's philosophy, the latter's defence of reason will play an important role in this chapter.

Critical self-reflection

In spite of the barbarity in which the enlightenment culminated, Adorno argues that we should try to cling to the basic promise of enlightenment thinking and stress the emancipatory qualities and possibilities of the faculty of reason. He and Horkheimer clearly state in the introduction to *Dialectic of Enlightenment*: 'We have no doubt – and herein lies our *petition principia* – that freedom in society is inseparable from enlightenment thinking.'[7] Immediately, however, the authors add the following to this statement:

> We believe we have perceived with equal clarity, however, that the very concept of that thinking, no less than the concrete historical forms, the institutions of society with which it is intertwined, already contains the germs of the regression which is taking place everywhere today. If enlightenment does not assimilate reflection on this regressive moment, it seals its own fate.[8]

This passage brings us to the first aspect of rationality that Adorno praises and that makes him different from Schopenhauer: the emancipating qualities of self-reflection and rational self-critique. Adorno often refers to Kant to illustrate the possibilities and capacities of this aspect of rationality. He observes in his lectures on *Problems of Moral Philosophy*, for example: 'A philosophy like Kant's ... never simply repeats what goes on in society, but has the tendency to criticize existing society and to hold up to it an alternative image of the possible, or an imageless image of the possible.'[9] In a sense, Adorno herewith returns to Kant's famous statement in the opening paragraph of 'An Answer to the Question: "What is Enlightenment?"':

> *Enlightenment is the human being's emergence from his self-incurred minority. Minority* is inability to make use of one's own understanding without direction from another. This minority is *self-incurred* when its cause is not in lack of understanding but in lack of resolution and courage to use it without direction from another. *Sapere aude!* Have courage to make use of your *own* understanding! is thus the motto of enlightenment.[10]

Adorno takes over Kant's emphasis on the critical aspects of enlightenment thinking, arguing that rational self-critique may enable us to see through the structures that guide our world and ourselves and look at the mechanisms behind them. These mechanisms may be based on tradition, on prejudices, on power, on historically developed discourses and ideologies, but also on drives and faculties within ourselves.

Adorno gives this idea a twist, however, by arguing that enlightenment thinking should be critical of *itself*, since – like every other tradition or discourse – it contains the tendency to transform into ideology; to overshadow the particular and thereby turn into the opposite of an open, free and critical approach to the world. In Chapter 5 we have seen that Adorno places this tendency in the constitution of a violent ego driven by self-preservation and argues that it has resulted, among other things, in a hostile approach towards everything different: in the Holocaust, in the culture industry and in the development of weapons of mass destruction. The ability to 'make use of one's own understanding' is therefore most of all obstructed by social structures and mechanisms, which means that a defence of enlightenment thought begins, in Adorno's view, with a critical analysis of socially and historically shaped ways of thinking.[11]

Adorno formulates this idea in *Negative Dialectics* as follows: 'critical self-reflection alone will keep [the subject ...] from building walls between itself and the object, from the supposition that its being-for-itself is an in-and-for-itself.'[12] In 'Education after Auschwitz', furthermore, he states:

> One must come to know the mechanisms that render people capable of such deeds [committing atrocities], must reveal these mechanisms to them, and strive, by awakening a general awareness of those mechanisms, to prevent people from becoming so again. ... The only education that has any sense at all is an education towards critical self-reflection.[13]

The tendency to identify the particular, to usurp the individual by subsuming it under broad categories and concepts and eventually to hurt it (as discussed in Chapter 5) might be tempered, in other words, by self-critique. The dialectical relationship between subject and object, between thought and its other, between concept and that which it tries to grasp, therefore needs to be negative in nature: the concept should not subsume the object it refers to, but keep itself at bay by reflecting on its own need to do this. In a dramatic passage, Adorno describes this process as follows:

> If negative dialectics calls for the self-reflection of thinking, the tangible implication is that if thinking is to be true – if it is to be true today, in any case – it must also be a thinking against itself. If thought is not measured by the extremity that eludes the concept, it is from the outset in the nature of the musical accompaniment with which the SS liked to drown out the screams of its victims.[14]

This emphasis on the critical capacities of reason suggests that Adorno does not completely reject rationality as a whole: even though he sometimes seems to argue that the faculty of reason is completely enslaved by a violent drive to self-preservation, he also claims that this situation is not so totalizingly grave that self-reflection is not possible anymore.

And even though the rational self has turned against itself in a hostile manner, Adorno places the ability to criticize this hostility in the origins of this same self. He writes in his lectures on *Problems of Moral Philosophy*: 'we are no longer simply a piece of nature from the moment we recognize we are a piece of nature.'[15] From the moment we realize on a reflective level that we *are* nature and that our rational thought is entwined with our nature as striving creatures, we have the key in our hands to partly pull ourselves out of the entwinement of nature and rationality by quietening down the drive to self-preservation, Adorno suggests. He describes this same idea in another characteristic phrase in his lectures on *History and Freedom*: 'absolute domination of nature is absolute submission to nature, and yet rises above nature when it reflects upon itself.'[16]

At the same time, however, the bleak nature of Adorno's diagnosis of the world forces him to claim that, even though the faculty of reason may provide us with the possibility to reflect, there are many social, cultural and historical factors that prevent us from doing precisely this.[17]

In the above-mentioned 'Education after Auschwitz', Adorno even mentions the Kantian notion of 'autonomy' as forming a key to the prevention of human catastrophes like Auschwitz:

> [T]he very willingness to connive with power and to submit outwardly to what is stronger, under the guise of a norm, is the attitude of the tormentors that should not arise again. It is for this reason that the advocacy of bonds is so fatal. People who adopt them more or less voluntarily are placed under a kind of permanent compulsion to obey orders. The single genuine power standing against the principle of Auschwitz is autonomy, if I might use the Kantian expression: the power of reflection, of self-determining, of not cooperating.[18]

It remains rather unclear, however, how Adorno believes this rational autonomy can be constituted: the observation that the rational subject may be able to reflect on itself does not mean that it has the capacity to change its own behaviour, to steer its own tendencies and to constitute this 'self-determinacy' Adorno refers to.

In Chapter 4, after all, we have seen that Schopenhauer emphasizes a similar capacity of the rational subject – the ability to analyse the mechanisms that steer its own behaviour, to realize that it is 'mauled as well as mauler' – *without* claiming that this capacity allows the subject to change its own behaviour. In Schopenhauer's philosophy, the rational subject is merely a powerless onlooker to its own enslavement. In order to differentiate his thought from Schopenhauer's and to counter Lukács and Habermas' observations that he reduces the subject to a similar passivity as Schopenhauer does, Adorno therefore has to do more than just emphasize the critical capacities of rationality.

The addendum and freedom

Social antinomy

This brings us to Adorno's analysis of the 'addendum' (*das Hinzutredende*). I want to discuss this complex concept by looking at his negative references to Kant: whereas we have seen above that he praises Kant's emphasis on critical self-reflection and autonomy, he criticizes him severely at other places. In the following, I want to show how and where Adorno's analysis of Kant's practical philosophy overlaps with Schopenhauer's. Since I am primarily concerned in this chapter with the similarities and differences between Schopenhauer and Adorno, I will not focus on ways in which Kant can be defended against their, at places, overly stereotypical interpretations. I return to this latter issue in Chapters 9 and 10.

In Chapter 5 I have shown that Adorno understands the modern subject as characterized by a pathological hostility against everything that is different. This hostility is driven by a rationality that is entwined with the drive to self-preservation and follows from an incorporation of social norms and mechanisms. Furthermore, it results in a self that is not only disconnected from the world and from other people but also from its own body. At several places Adorno links these observations to an interpretation of the Kantian transcendental self and approaches Kant's philosophy as a reflection of the dominating nature of the faculty of reason.

Adorno mainly criticizes Kant's philosophy for its 'exclusion of all desires and impulses'[19] and portrays his emphasis on rational self-constitution as the triumph of a violently repressive super-ego over anything that borders on the body, impulsivity or sensuality, instrumentalizing, controlling and mechanizing the corporeal dimension of human existence and making it into a 'static' and 'sanitized' object. The Kantian self – more accurately: that which it embodies, in Adorno's view – is encapsulated in its own self-declared autonomy: 'Kant's Copernican turn precisely expresses the objectification of the subject'.[20] Adorno is specifically concerned with the possibility of freedom in this context: '[Kant's] philosophy starts off by postulating freedom and extracts an immense pathos from it, but in the process of developing its meaning, this freedom dwindles to the point of extinction and his philosophy ends up by dispensing with freedom entirely'.[21]

This brings us back to Schopenhauer's analysis of Kant's theory of action. In Chapter 4 we have seen that the former criticizes the latter's dichotomy between the intelligible and the practical realms: in Schopenhauer's view, the subject is not able to bridge the gap between these two realms and can therefore only be thought of as free once it is completely passive and remains within the intelligible realm, or as unfree once it acts and manifests itself as an embodied subject in the practical realm. Every act, Schopenhauer concludes, is part of a chain of cause and effect and therefore determined: the acting self is unfree. Schopenhauer furthermore claims that he arrives at this conclusion because he takes Kant's philosophy to its logical extreme; even though he himself, as we have seen, was not able to develop a satisfying theory about the connection between the intelligible and the practical character either.

A similar point about Kant's philosophy is made by Adorno. Given Kant's characterizations of the empirical character on the one hand and the intelligible character on the other, Adorno observes that we are unable to conceptualize an *active* being in the *intelligible* realm or a *free* being in the *empirical* realm. As Schopenhauer already discussed, Adorno observes that a person can only be active once it crosses the divide between the intelligible and the practical realms; once the purely rational subject manages to constitute itself as an acting self *in* the empirical world. However, if we argue that this happens through causality, that the intelligible character, in some way or another, *leaps* to the empirical world by *causing* an act, this act becomes part of the world of the senses and the intelligible character is drawn into the empirical world, which is a world in which freedom does not exist:

> While Kant, in practical philosophy, rigorously proclaims the *chorismos* of what is and what ought to be, he is nonetheless compelled to resort to mediations. His idea of freedom turns into a paradox: it comes to be incorporated in the causality of the phenomenal world that is incompatible with the Kantian concept of freedom.[22]

In the first model in *Negative Dialectics* Adorno argues that Kant tried to solve this problem by relying on the notion of 'will': 'It is through the will, [Kant] says, that reason creates its reality, untrammelled by the material, whatever its kind.'[23] But by defining this will as 'a sort of causality of living creatures, provided they are rational', the concept of 'will', Adorno claims, 'becomes a no-man's-land between subject and object'[24] and 'owes its plausibility solely to the abstraction which has reason exhaust the will without a remainder'.[25] By introducing the notion of 'will', in other words, Kant seeks to infuse the rational self with *force*, with a *spontaneity* that allows us to explain the coming about of an act in the empirical world. However, by claiming at the same time that this will is completely devoid of anything sensual, of any kind of material impulsivity, we end up with a force that cannot be thought of as a force, but floats in a vacuum between the intelligible and the empirical realms.[26]

In *Negative Dialectics* Adorno therefore approaches Schopenhauer's theory regarding the unfreedom of the self as reflecting the wrongness of Kant's rationalism: 'What the great rationalistic philosophers conceived as the will is already, and without accounting for it, a denial of the will. The Schopenhauer of Book Four had every right to feel that he was a Kantian.'[27] In the fourth book of *The World as Will and Representation*, Schopenhauer discusses his ideas on denying and overcoming the will, to which I return in Chapter 9. Schopenhauer's theory, in other words, forms a parody of Kant's inability to reconcile the acting self with the rational self, Adorno argues, and shows us that the notion of willing eventually dissolves in Kant's rationalism.

Unlike Schopenhauer, Adorno does not want to conclude that the acting subject is completely unfree, determined by a world permeated with causality. At the same time, however, he understands Kant's dichotomy between the intelligible and practical realms and especially its hostility towards embodiment as reflecting a truth moment about the historical situation he criticizes. The unfreedom that the self has in a world defined by causality, in other words, reflects the unfreedom that characterizes life in a social whole in which individuals are reduced to mere cogs in a machine and in which they have developed a distant and cold relationship with their own bodies. In *Negative Dialectics* Adorno therefore criticizes Kant as follows: 'The imprisonment in immanence to which [Kant] honestly and brutally condemns the mind is the imprisonment in self-preservation, as it is imposed on men by a society that conserves nothing but denials that would not be necessary anymore.'[28] Kant's antinomy, in Adorno's view, reflects an objective, social antinomy, and his understanding of a gap between the intelligible and the practical realms reflects the wrongness of a world in which the self is unable to freely manifest itself as an embodied, autonomous being.

The addendum

In light of these two observations, Adorno seeks to develop an understanding of what acting is and, eventually, what freedom entails without naively stepping over this dichotomy altogether and ignoring the grimness of the historical situation that he finds embodied by Kant's works and parodied by Schopenhauer's.

It is within this context that he introduces the concept of the addendum, which he describes as follows:

> To philosophical reflection [the addendum] appears as downright otherness because the will that has been reduced to pure practical

> reason is an abstraction. The addendum is the name for that which was eliminated in this abstraction; without it, there would be no real will at all. It is a flash of light between the poles of something long past, something grown all but unrecognizable, and that which some day might come to be.[29]

Placed within the dichotomy between subject and object, the addendum forms a rather ungraspable and mysterious element that combines both the subjective world and the material world and creates the possibility of a mind, of *subjectivity*, to manifest itself in the world, in *objectivity*, through bodily acts. It is this element, in other words, that links the *a priori* and the *a posteriori*; that forms the connection between mind and body within Adorno's analysis. Espen Hammer helpfully defines this 'physical moment'[30] as 'a rather mysterious anarchic other than reason'.[31]

To a certain extent, these characterizations of the addendum are similar to Adorno's observations developed in *Against Epistemology*, discussed in Chapter 2. We have there seen that he argues that the subject needs a material kind of 'friction', a bodily form of contact with the world – a 'bit of nature'[32] – in order to have experiences of this world at all. The notion of a purely transcendental or purely rational subject, he observes, cannot make sense of perception because it overlooks the body.

In his lectures on *History and Freedom*, Adorno argues that Shakespeare's *Hamlet* provides us with an illustration of the addendum: Hamlet famously needs an external impulse to act (the infliction of a wound). He needs to be *infused* with energy to break through the immanence of his subjectivity; to tear down the fossilized walls around his ego and to manifest himself 'in the world' as an acting being.[33]

The introduction of this element makes it possible for Adorno, in contrast with Schopenhauer, to argue that critical self-reflection may play an active role and temper or confront certain drives and tendencies within the self. By introducing the addendum, a bodily and spontaneous impulse, in other words, Adorno seeks to evade the above-mentioned 'imprisonment in immanence' to which Kant condemns the rational self, and to connect this self to its body.

In Chapters 3 and 4 I have argued that one of the most important and unique aspects of Schopenhauer's theory of the primacy of Will is his idea that body and mind are entwined and that we are dependent on materialistic processes and conditions over which we do not have complete rational control. In a more subtle way, aspects of this idea echo through Adorno's discussion of the addendum. He writes in *Negative Dialectics*:

> Though the addendum may always be more sublimated with increasing consciousness, though indeed the concept of the will as something substantial and anonymous may only be formed in that increase – if the motor form of reaction were liquidated altogether, if the hand no longer twitched, there would be no will.[34]

Descriptions like these hint at the following five characteristics of the addendum. First, the addendum contains irrational elements, since it cannot be entirely defined by the realm of the rational. This, after all, is one of the main points of critique Adorno formulates against Kant. Second, the addendum contains a materialistic element but, third, is not *completely* materialistic either. It exists on the border between body and psyche, being neither unmediated corporeal instinct, nor rational and deliberate action. Indeed, Adorno observes, again in *Negative Dialectics*, that the concept of the addendum 'denies the Cartesian dualism of *res extensa* and *res cogitans*'[35] and that it is 'intramental and somatic in one'.[36] In his lectures on *History and Freedom*, furthermore, he states that it is 'both somatic and mental at the same time'.[37] The addendum should therefore be interpreted along psychoanalytic lines as existing on the border between body and psyche, being neither unmediated corporeal instinct nor rational and deliberate action, but a *drive* that constitutes one's will.[38]

The fourth characteristic of the addendum is that it has a social and critical dimension: the divide between subject and object is understood as reflecting a historical situation, which suggests that the gap between subject and object, mind and body, has not always been as wide as Adorno observes. He indeed defines the addendum as 'an impulse, the rudiment of a phase in which the dualism of extramental and intramental was not thoroughly consolidated yet, neither volitively bridgeable nor an ontological ultimate'.[39]

A fifth characteristic relates to these last two observations: the addendum is *itself* embedded in a historical context, which implies that the ways in which we experience our bodies, including our impulses and needs, are influenced by the culture in which we live. Unlike Schopenhauer, who claims that we are simply overcome by instincts that we share with all living creatures (human and non-human), Adorno makes room, for example, for the idea that people who live in different cultures and different times may experience their sexuality and their corporeality in different ways.

In his article on Adorno and Freud, Whitebook compares Adorno with the founder of psychoanalysis in a passage that I want to cite here because it characterizes the relation between Adorno and Schopenhauer's thought as well. Whitebook argues that Adorno's claim in *Dialectic of Enlightenment* that the body forms a 'subterranean history' of Europe – discussed in Chapter 5 – refers not to the 'natural body', but contains a Foucauldian reading of the body as the nexus of social and discursive forms of power and is therefore based on a historification of classical psychoanalysis: 'Almost unnoticed', Whitebook writes, '*the constructed body has been slipped in to replace the material body.* This substitution is motivated by an understandable desire to replace Freud's perceived biologism, which would condemn us to an immutable essentialism in sexual matters, with constructivism.'[40]

Freedom and rationality

This discussion of the addendum provides us with a better idea of Adorno's position on rationality. First, he claims that reason is always entwined with embodiment, with impulsivity, and therefore contains irrational elements. On the one hand, he approaches this as a rather obvious observation that applies to everyone who tries to think about action in purely rational terms: his analysis of Kant's ideas on action suggests that we can never think about a purely rational subject without there being a 'physical remainder'. On the other hand, his grim diagnosis of the status quo is mainly based on the idea that rationality is entwined with the drive to self-preservation, which means that besides being a theoretical observation about action, it also contains a pessimistic diagnosis of a historical age.

Second, Adorno claims that the experience we have of our bodies is always permeated with historical categories and influenced by the culture in which we live. On the one hand, he approaches this observation again as a rather obvious analysis of the nature of culture, but understands its results on the other as underlying one of the bleak aspects of modernity – we have seen that he criticizes the culture industry for 'desexualizing' sexuality.[41]

Furthermore, the fact that Adorno bases the ability to act on an addendum, on a remainder, on a spark that refuses to be rationalized away, means that the historical context in which he develops this analysis has become so wrong, in his view, that it completely distorts the balance between body and mind. The latter pole of this relationship can only be referred to vaguely, since otherwise it would immediately be included in a way of thinking that robs it of that which makes it into 'the other' of the mind, he suggests: its non-conceptual, partly irrational and ungraspable nature. The addendum has been reduced to what he calls 'the twitching of the hand'; to a bodily reflex over which one has almost no control. Within modernity, in other words, freedom can only be understood as a brief moment that is almost completely overshadowed by wrongness. In *Negative Dialectics* he summarizes these ideas as follows: 'Freedom is a moment…in a twofold sense: it is entwined, not to be isolated; and for the time being it is never more than an instant of spontaneity, a historical node, the road to which is blocked under present conditions.'[42]

Conclusion

In contrast with Lukács and Habermas' critical analyses of Adorno's thought and its, in their views, nihilistic approach to rationality, I have shown that his works do contain positive references to the faculty of reason. It is true, however, that his analysis of the abilities of the rational subject to act rests on rather obscure references to a vague bodily spark that is, in his own view, almost completely overshadowed by a false whole.

Furthermore, the observation that Adorno's works are so negative that they hardly leave open the possibility of referring to the modern subject in a positive manner, do make his diagnosis of the status quo border on the pessimistic views of Schopenhauer. Nevertheless, these thinkers are not the same and Adorno provides us with a more constructive, subtle and historically relevant notion of rationality than Schopenhauer, according to whom there is no hope for the rational self.

The differences between both follow mainly from the historical twist Adorno gives to his analysis of the self's powerlessness. Even though the ideas of both originate in a similar critical reading of Kant, Adorno distinguishes his ideas on freedom from Schopenhauer's in several respects. First, the observation that every subject is always entwined with the culture and society in which it grows up does not mean that it is by definition unfree. This is only the case under the specific historical conditions Adorno criticizes. In different social circumstances, in other words, freedom might be found. Adorno therefore argues against Kant – and this argument could be directed at Schopenhauer as well – that freedom 'might be essentially historic'.[43]

Second, Adorno's observation that people understand themselves as autarkic is not an ahistorical given either: again, it follows from historical ways of thinking among which, for example, the idea prevails that individuals should compete with each other and are only responsible for their own well-being.

Third, Adorno suggests that freedom can be found precisely when people realize that they *are* part of social conditions and that they should change these same conditions in order to better the quality of their lives.[44] Instead of covering one's eyes with the veil of Maya, claiming that one is absolutely independent and that every individual is responsible for his or her own well-being – the situation Adorno defines as 'cold' – Adorno suggests that one might find freedom precisely on the crossing point between self and society, realizing that absolute autonomy and absolute freedom are illusory and ideological concepts.

Autonomy is found, in other words, if one does not obsessively or neurotically seek to distance oneself from the cultural and social whole in which one lives or from the body that one has, but if one recognizes one's dependence on processes that may not be entirely rational. I develop these observations further in Chapters 8 and 10.

Part II

Morality, Salvation, Happiness

7
Neminem Laede – Injure No One

Introduction

In the second excursus of *Dialectic of Enlightenment* Max Horkheimer approaches the literary universe developed in the novels of the Marquis de Sade as the embodiment of the instrumental rationality he and Adorno saw arising with the birth of the modern self. In his analysis of Sade's writings, Horkheimer refers to a philosophical problem that, as I will argue in this and the following chapters, follows from both Schopenhauer and Adorno's works: how are we able to develop a sound normative basis of morality if the whole in which this is attempted is characterized as 'wrong' – at places even as 'evil' – and if the human subject embedded in this whole is claimed to have very little control over its actions?

The worldview of Juliette, which Horkheimer equates with the worldview of 'radical enlightenment',[1] eradicates the possibility of referring to feelings like warmth, love, care, compassion, solidarity or tenderness. Furthermore, the faculty of reason is deemed to have no other role than piercing through the sentimentality and relativity of moral philosophies. In *Justine*, for example, we find the following passage on murder:

> [T]his crime, which you find so enormous, is really, at bottom, a very simple thing.... As far as the destruction of one's kind is concerned, you may be certain... that such a belief is entirely chimerical, since the power of destruction has not been accorded to man. At the very most he has the ability of causing things to change form – but he cannot annihilate them.... And of what importance is it to eternally creative nature, if this mass of flesh which today presents the shape of a woman, should tomorrow reproduce itself in the guise of a thousand different insects?[2]

Emotions are fleeting and powerless, mere sentimentality, Sade suggests, and our faculty of reason only confirms the observation that the world is a meaningless whole, consisting of a blind nature that is as cruel as it is nihilistic. This means that both reason and emotions are, in his view, unable to form or construct a normative basis of moral thought.

These ideas come very close to the pessimistic conclusions that follow from Schopenhauer's metaphysics of Will: if everything is driven by a blind force, manifesting itself as a drive to self-preservation or a need to procreate, and if human beings have no rational control over that which drives them, then what role is left for a moral philosophy to play? Does morality not disappear once the subject is believed to be completely overshadowed by the metaphysical and unchangeable essence of the universe, and reduced to a mere cog in a metaphysical machine?

In this chapter I will focus on this question and show how Schopenhauer tries to translate his observations on Will, compassion and rationality into a normative basis of moral thought.

Practical reason and Will

A theological ought

Schopenhauer shapes his moral philosophy against the horizon of Kant's ideas on practical reason. I therefore first want to look at the precise ways in which he criticizes Kant's moral theory before evaluating his own ideas on morality.

As discussed in Chapter 4, Schopenhauer's observations on volition and agency revolve around the idea that human beings have no rational control over that which they do. He mainly bases this conclusion on a critique of Kant's analysis of the intelligible and practical characters and, more specifically, of his inability (in Schopenhauer's view) to include the acting body in this dichotomy: the subject, Schopenhauer observes, cannot be free and, at the same time, constitute itself as an acting creature in a practical realm defined by causality. Taking over Kant's dichotomy, Schopenhauer concludes that the subject is unfree and has no control over that which it does.

Entering the realm of morality, this observation corrodes the foundation and possibility of Kant's categorical imperative as follows: since reason, in Schopenhauer's view, is not able to motivate human beings, he accuses Kant of developing a moral theology that is based on an 'ought' that is never experienced as an 'ought' in itself: it merely forms a remainder of a theological morality that *used to* be motivating because it was based on the ideas of divine punishment and divine approval: 'separated from the theological hypotheses from which they came, these concepts really lose all meaning, and when anyone like Kant imagines he can substitute those hypotheses by speaking of absolute ought and unconditioned duty, he is feeding the reader on fair words.'[3]

Since human beings are not motivated by reason but by the drives, feelings and emotions that make up someone's unchangeable character, Schopenhauer argues, we have to conclude that Kant either defends an empty and powerless formalistic philosophy or secretly relies on subjective needs – like selfishness and egotism – as drives motivated by moral ideas. Kant's unconditional norms only gain a motivating quality, in other words, if the subject *fears* divine punishment or *needs* the idea of a benevolent afterlife: only then are these norms able to trigger the empirical and unchangeable character of an individual and bring about a bodily act. Schopenhauer writes:

> Just as we know *intelligence in general* to be an attribute simply and solely of animal beings, and are therefore never justified in thinking of it as existing outside and independent of animal nature, so do we know *reason* (Vernunft) as the exclusive attribute of the human race, and are by no means entitled to think of it as existing outside that race, and to set up a *genus* called 'rational beings' differing from its sole species, 'man.' Still less are we justified in laying down laws for such imaginary *rational beings in the abstract*. To talk of rational beings apart from man is as if we attempted to talk of *heavy beings* apart from bodies.[4]

Kant defends a morality that applies to a type of person that does not exist, in Schopenhauer's view: a purely rational being and, as his metaphor in the last line of the cited passage illustrates, a being without a body, without gravity, without a carnal dimension; an *immaterial* being that originates in the (theological) idea that the 'immaterial' and rational 'soul' is a 'high' capacity that conflicts with 'low' desires and needs, Schopenhauer observes.[5]

In defence of Kant

It could be argued that Schopenhauer's critique is based on an overly stereotypical interpretation of Kant's moral philosophy. For example, he seems to overlook the idea that Kant aims at actions that purely rational beings *would* do, thereby developing a highly critical theory about what human beings *actually* do.[6] Claiming that Kant's understanding of practical reason is not realistic misses the point that its unrealistic nature is what makes it into a highly critical morality. In Chapter 6 we have seen that Adorno praises precisely this aspect of Kant's philosophy because it holds up to existing society 'an alternative image of the possible, or an imageless image of the possible.'[7]

However, we have seen as well that Adorno claims that the idea of a completely rational subject is a myth and that, once we conceptualize the acting self in purely rational terms, there will always be a bodily remainder: the addendum. Like Schopenhauer, Adorno suggests that Kant's moral philosophy does not revolve around that which most people *could* do and do not *actually* do, but around an idea of human action that is, *by definition*, unrealistic.

It has also been argued that Schopenhauer's critique misses the point that Kant does not merely seek to critically 'unleash' reason but, especially in his first *Critique*, precisely tries to set limits to the role rationality can and should play, thereby defining and securing the freedom that the rational subject is able to find.[8] Again, however, in Adorno's works we find the claim that even though this may have been the initial idea behind Kant's philosophy, this does not mean that Kant's project did not eventually turn into a celebration of the dominating qualities of rationality: '[Kant's] philosophy starts off by postulating freedom and extracts an immense pathos from it, but in the process of developing its meaning, this freedom dwindles to the point of extinction and his philosophy ends up by dispensing with freedom entirely.'[9]

Even though I think that both authors make use of a quite stereotypical reading of Kant, in which the subtleties of the latter's philosophy are lost, the scope of this chapter does not allow me to discuss the intricacies of the ways in which Kant can be defended against Schopenhauer's (and Adorno's) critique. I want to argue, however, that it is important to take the observation into account that both Schopenhauer and Adorno are more concerned with that which Kant's philosophy *represents* than with that which it precisely says. For Schopenhauer, Kant's thought embodies the ideas of absolute autonomy and rational self-control, of enlightenment optimism and hope in the emancipatory qualities of the human self. For Adorno, it embodies the socially conditioned repression of everything bodily by a hostile and instrumentalized faculty of reason that proclaims complete control over that which it seeks to grasp.

In the following, I want to follow up on this idea by showing that we find several interesting arguments in Schopenhauer's works against a moral philosophy that is completely rational in nature. I will thereby emphasize the strength of his arguments, which mainly revolve around the phenomena of compassion and bodily pain, by confronting them with Christine Korsgaard's moral philosophy. In Chapter 8 I return to Adorno's critique of Kant and to his own contribution to moral philosophy.

Compassion and suffering

Against normativity

Most explicitly in his 1840 work *On the Basis of Morality*, but also in the essay 'On Ethics' in *Parerga and Paralipomena*, in the chapter 'Reference to Ethics' in *On the Will in Nature*, and in the fourth book of *The World as Will and Representation*, Schopenhauer discusses the normative basis of morality. It would be wrong, however, to conclude that the sphere of the moral is restricted to these parts of his oeuvre; most of his works are permeated with and originate in a moral concern with the well-being of other creatures – both human and non-human.[10] In Chapter 3, for example, we have seen that Schopenhauer claims that 'the only Metaphysics which really and immediately supports Ethics, is that one which is itself primarily ethical and constituted out of the material of Ethics'.[11]

Based on his critique of Kant and the idea of a purely rational acting self in general, Schopenhauer draws the quite radical conclusion that moral philosophy has no prescribing function at all, only a descriptive one, and provides his essay 'On the basis of morality' with the following motto 'To preach morality is easy, to found it difficult'.[12] Since human beings have no rational control over their actions they are not able to wilfully submit themselves to a rational law or to change their behaviour in order to conform to a moral system, he argues: 'We should...be just as foolish to expect that our moral systems and ethics would create virtuous, noble and holy men, as that our aesthetics would produce poets, painters, and musicians.'[13] In *On the Basis of Morality* Schopenhauer defines the methodological framework of his analysis of morality as follows:

> I shall probably be told that ethics is not concerned with how people actually behave, but that it is the science that states how they *ought* to behave. But this is the very principle which I deny, after showing clearly enough...that the concept of ought, the imperative form of ethics, applies solely to theological morality, and that outside this it loses all sense and meaning. I assume, on the other hand, that

> the purpose of ethics is to indicate, explain, and trace to its ultimate ground the extremely varied behavior of men from a moral point of view. Therefore there is no other way for discovering the foundation of ethics than the empirical, namely, to investigate whether there are generally any actions to which we must attribute *genuine moral worth*.... This is the humble path to which I direct ethics: it contains no construction a priori, no absolute legislation for all rational beings *in abstracto*.[14]

Not only does this claim find its theoretical basis in Schopenhauer's understanding of motivation and psychology as discussed in Chapter 4, it is also based on the more pragmatic observation that in difficult situations no one turns towards a rational norm or law in order to decide what to do: 'Morality', he writes, 'is concerned with the actual conduct of man, and not with the a priori building of houses of cards to whose results no man would turn in the storm and stress of life.'[15]

Compassion

This brings us to the phenomenon of compassion with suffering creatures, which Schopenhauer understands as the ground of behaviour we call 'moral'. As we have seen in Chapter 2, Schopenhauer's struggles with epistemology culminate in an antinomy between a world dependent on the perceiving subject on the one hand and a perceiving subject embedded in the material world on the other. I have argued that it is his concern with the body that makes him end up in this paradoxical epistemological position, which returns in both Merleau-Ponty's *Phenomenology of Perception* and in Adorno's *Against Epistemology*, although in different forms. This same concern with corporeality underlies Schopenhauer's metaphysics, which he bases on the idea that the body provides us with a key to the essence of the universe and which revolves around several contradictions caused by his analysis of embodiment. His moral philosophy is born of a similar focus on the realm of the somatic: it is based on the idea that the suffering of our fellow creatures is wrong and that we should do anything in our power to prevent it. Schopenhauer observes: 'there is an analogy between what is moral and what is physiological.'[16]

This sensitivity to suffering can be traced back to an experience Schopenhauer had when he was seventeen years old. At that age, he witnessed the suffering of galley-slaves in the dungeons of Toulon and wrote in his diary about the profound impact it made on him.[17] This experience can be understood as one of the first real confrontations

Schopenhauer had with the barbarity that humanity is capable of. It triggered the idea in him that the world may not be designed for the well-being of those that live in it, and that human beings are not the moral creatures they are often portrayed to be. As mentioned in the Introduction to this book, the example of slavery indeed returns several times in his work as an example of the evil that human beings are capable of doing to their fellow human beings. In *Parerga and Paralipomena*, for example, we find a vicious attack on the manner in which 'those devils in human form, those bigoted, church-going, strict Sabbath-observing scoundrels, especially the Anglican parsons among them, treat their innocent black brothers who through violence and injustice have fallen into their devils' claws'.[18]

This response of abhorrence, felt whilst witnessing the suffering of the galley-slaves, can be understood as a prime example of the phenomenon that forms the core of Schopenhauer's descriptive moral philosophy: compassion. Only the occurrence of compassion, Schopenhauer argues, may be able to counter the feelings of egotism that, more often than not, define the behaviour of human beings.

In Chapter 3 we have seen that Schopenhauer embeds compassion in his metaphysics: since everything, essentially, is a manifestation of an in-itself that knows no *principium individuationis*, we are all unified on a metaphysical level and therefore able to experience the suffering of other creatures 'in' ourselves. He links these metaphysical observations to his moral philosophy as follows:

> The process here analysed is not one that is imagined or invented; on the contrary it is perfectly real and indeed by no means infrequent. It is the everyday phenomenon of *compassion*, of the immediate *participation*, independent of all ulterior considerations, primarily in the *suffering* of another, and thus in the prevention or elimination of it; for all satisfaction and all well-being and happiness consist in this. It is simply and solely this compassion that is the real basis of all voluntary justice and genuine loving-kindness.[19]

Suffering should be prevented, Schopenhauer claims, and it is not a rationally constructed rule or a divine law that tells us so but feelings of compassion with our fellow creatures.

Since his moral theory is completely descriptive in nature, Schopenhauer suggests that we cannot explain *why* pain is wrong or *why* the suffering of both ourselves and others should be prevented. He only observes that pain is experienced negatively by creatures that are vulnerable to suffering: once we experience it, we want it to go away. And once we are confronted with the pain of others through the phenomenon of compassion, we want their suffering to be over as quickly as possible as well (as long as we are not overpowered by egotistic tendencies).

The only reason Schopenhauer provides for the observation that pain is unpleasant is the claim that it confronts the Will, as discussed in Chapter 4.[20] However, this is only an explanation and not a rationally developed argument for *why* pain is bad or what norms or ideas it goes against. In that same chapter, I have argued that this idea forms one of the pillars on which Schopenhauer's pessimism rests. When confronted with the suffering that takes place in the world, he observes, we instinctively reject the conditions under which this happens and the world in which this takes place: 'If we were to conduct the most hardened and callous optimist through hospitals, infirmaries, operating theatres, through prisons, torture-chambers, and slave-hovels, over battlefields and to places of execution ... he too would certainly see in the end what kind of a world is this *meilleur des mondes possibles*.'[21] As Volker Spierling states in his introduction to Schopenhauer's lectures on the *Metaphysik der Sitten*: 'Schopenhauer ... stellt der Philosophie den Schmerz des Leibes in den Weg.'[22]

The normativity of pain

Different kinds of pain

In order to shed light on these rather bold and not unproblematic statements, I want to compare Schopenhauer's observations on pain and compassion with those developed by Christine Korsgaard, whose theory of rational endorsement I analysed in Chapter 4 in the context of Schopenhauer's ideas on rationality and self-constitution.

As discussed, Korsgaard argues that normativity arises the moment one reflects on oneself as a rational being, which forces one to rationally decide which ends one wants to set oneself. And these ends only become binding once they conform to the *a priori* norms and values one has set oneself from a rational point of view.

Korsgaard therefore rejects the idea that pain and suffering carry a normative value on their own, as Schopenhauer's above-cited observations suggest. She thereby mainly criticizes David Hume, who famously argued in a rather Schopenhauerian fashion that 'reason is, and ought only to be the slave of the passions, and can never pretend to any other office than to serve and obey them.'[23] In a passage that could have been written by Schopenhauer, Hume therefore writes the following about Cicero condemning the crimes of Verres or Catiline:

> The orator may paint rage, insolence, barbarity on the one side: Meekness, suffering, sorrow, innocence on the other: But if you feel no indignation or compassion arise in you from this complication of circumstances, you would in vain ask him, in what consists the crime of villainy, which he so vehemently exclaims against:... No satisfactory answer can be given... upon the abstract hypothesis of morals: and we must at last acknowledge, that the crime or immorality is no particular fact or relation, which can be the object of the understanding: But arises entirely from the sentiment of disapprobation, which, by the structure of human nature, we unavoidably feel on the apprehension of barbarity or treachery.[24]

Following her notion of rational endorsement, discussed in Chapter 4, Korsgaard criticizes Hume for developing the idea that 'pleasure and pain are facts which are also values, a place where the natural and normative are one, and so where ethics can find a foundation in the natural world'.[25] If this would be the case, the *reason* for endorsing certain incentives – for example, our rejection of the pain of other beings – would not originate in its conformation with a rationally and *a priori* constructed principle.

Korsgaard therefore claims in *The Sources of Normativity*, contra Hume, that pain is not, simply, an animalistic *response* to a situation. One of her reasons for this claim is the strong observation that even though pain is in most cases bad, it is not *intrinsically bad* from a moral point of view. She provides the following two examples:

> First, we don't always object to the sensations that we sometimes call 'pain'. An acute sensation, say, of effort or of appetite will be welcome in one context, unwelcome in another.... And sometimes we welcome, not just the sensations to which in other contexts we object, but even pain itself. No one, I suppose, would choose not to experience grief at the death of a loved one at all, although we are rightly afraid of finding it unbearable.[26]

It could be argued from a physiological point of view that 'all pain is intrinsically bad': our bodies respond to pain in a negative way. Whether I hurt myself in a car accident, accidently cut my finger when I'm making a sandwich, experience pain when my dentist is filling a hole in my teeth, or suffer when I'm being tortured, my body responds in a negative way.

But there is more to pain than physiological impact alone, Korsgaard argues, since we embed it in the context in which we experience it. For example, if I experience pain when my dentist is pulling one of my teeth, I evaluate this pain in light of the knowledge that it will lead to good results in the future, even though the bodily experience of the pain *itself* is negative. In other words: whereas it could be claimed that 'all pain is bad' on the level of physical reactions, the term 'badness' does, on this level, not have a *moral* meaning.

This is a strong argument against descriptive moral philosophies like Hume's and Schopenhauer's, especially since Schopenhauer himself makes a similar distinction between different kinds of pain: he only judges *certain* forms of pain to be wrong from a moral point of view and even refers positively to specific forms of suffering.

An example can be found in his discussion of the role that suffering plays in the life of saints. I extensively return to this aspect of his philosophy in Chapter 9, which revolves around his ideas on self-denial, but in the context of our current discussion it is relevant to mention that Schopenhauer refers several times to suffering in a positive manner. He argues, for example, that pain can strengthen the 'life-denier' in his or her eventual turning away from the world and writes about 'suffering and dying becoming agreeable' once 'the denial of the will-to-live has made its appearance', observing about the experience of salvation: 'It is the gleam of silver that suddenly appears from the purifying flame of suffering, the gleam of the denial of the will-to-live, of salvation.'[27]

These claims regarding the 'purifying flame of suffering' influence our analysis of the normative basis of Schopenhauer's moral philosophy. Whereas we may have the *same* initial and *causal* bodily response of shock when we perceive, for example, an Indian *sadhu* who pierces his own body with knives in order to gain enlightenment, someone who gets stabbed in a fight, or a soldier whose wounds are treated without anaesthetics because he will otherwise die, Schopenhauer makes room for the observation that our moral judgement of each of these situations is different.

This does not mean however, and this is a very important point, that the *why* behind these moral judgements is, eventually, rational in nature. Even though we may choose to accept pain in one situation and reject it in another, it could still be argued from a Schopenhauerian point of view that this evaluative decision is based on the attempt to prevent more pain in the future or to increase my eventual well-being.

The normative grounds on which my judgement of these different kinds of pain are based, in other words, do not have to be rational but may still very well lie in my initial experience of pain as bad, something that I cannot further ground rationally. Even though I may be able to create a reflective distance between myself and my feelings and responses, overlook the future and decide which pains I endorse and which I reject, the arguments that I use to make this decision might very well refer back to my initial, instinctive and negative responses to pain.[28]

Animal suffering and compassion

This brings us back to Korsgaard's analysis of pain. What makes pain into a challenging example is that non-human animals experience pain as well and, like human animals, have a tendency to avoid it. In Chapter 3 we have seen that Schopenhauer indeed includes non-human animals in his moral philosophy.[29]

This introduces the problematic question whether non-human animals *endorse* pain as a *reason* before they act in response to it *or* whether there is a fundamental difference between the way human and non-human animals experience pain. Korsgaard answers this question as follows:

> A living thing is an entity whose nature it is to preserve and maintain its physical identity. It is a law to itself. When something it is doing is a threat to that identity and perception reveals that fact, the animal finds that it must reject what it is doing and do something else instead. In that case, it is in pain. Obligation is the reflective rejection of a threat to your identity. Pain is the *unreflective* rejection of a threat to your identity. So pain is the *perception* of a reason, and that is why it seems so normative.[30]

In Korsgaard's view, pleasure and pain are therefore 'expressive of the value that an animal places on itself',[31] which means the following: 'An animal which is in pain is objecting to its condition. But it also objects to being in a condition to which it objects.'[32]

In her essay 'From Duty and for the Sake of the Noble: Kant and Aristotle on Morally Good Action', Korsgaard shifts from a first-person to a third-person perspective and struggles with this same problem regarding the notion of 'sympathy'. Since we, in most cases, reject the pain of others in a rather instinctive manner like we would reject our own pain, she approaches these two phenomena from the same angle and even includes, as does Schopenhauer, compassion with non-human animals in her analysis.[33] She does this by asserting, in analogy to her interpretation of pain, that she takes 'our natural sympathy with the other animals ... to be perceptions of the reasons we have to be merciful and protective towards them'.[34]

Trying to take our feelings of sympathy and compassion with human and non-human animals seriously, Korsgaard herewith rejects Kant's exclusive focus on rationality. In *Groundwork of the Metaphysics of Morals*, after all, Kant famously stated:

> To be beneficent where one can is one's duty, and besides there are many souls so attuned to compassion that, even without another motivating ground of vanity, or self-interest, they find an inner gratification in spreading joy around them, and can relish the contentment of others, in so far as it is their work. But I assert that in such a case an action of this kind – however much it conforms with duty, however amiable it may be – still has no true moral worth, but stands on the same footing as other inclinations.[35]

Korsgaard responds to Kant as follows:

> Kant cannot see natural sympathy as an inchoate grasp of the fact that there is a reason to help. He thinks that an inclination signals only a certain subjective suitability between the sympathetic person and the promotion of the happiness of others, a fitness of sympathetic action to gratify this particular person.... For Kant, sympathy is not a proto-virtue but merely a kind of substitute for virtue which nature has given us in the meantime.[36]

Korsgaard, in other words, disagrees with Kant and argues that our ability to experience compassion with suffering others already grants us with a *reason* to base moral behaviour on.

The truth moment of Korsgaard's moral philosophy

This raises the question, however, of whether Korsgaard's understanding of the 'perception of a reason' is that different from the instrumental role that rationality plays in Schopenhauer's moral philosophy. By understanding pain and sympathy with beings that are in pain as perceptions of a reason that can be both conscious and unconscious in nature, Korsgaard departs quite drastically from her initially Kantian approach to rationality and pulls her understanding of what rational endorsement means back into the realm of nature. By arguing that an animal does not avoid pain because this pain hurts but because the animal *perceives* that that which it *values* is in danger – its identity[37] – and that this same mechanism underlies our rejection of the pain of *other* beings, I believe that Korsgaard ends up with a rather instrumental understanding of what rational endorsement means.

By describing pain and suffering in this way, Korsgaard furthermore shifts from a moral philosophy that is normative, that provides us with guiding principles that enable us to decide which norms we seek to follow, to a more *descriptive* theory that analyses what both human and non-human animals do when they experience pain.

Like Schopenhauer, she argues that the self does not endorse a desire or impulse *from a rational point of view* in the Kantian sense – that is, because this desire or impulse is endorsed by a rationally constructed principle – but claims that this endorsement 'happens' by *perceiving* something *as a reason*, something that animals are capable of as well. Like Schopenhauer, she thus argues that we have the ability to make normative distinctions between different kinds of pain, even to argue why certain types of suffering are beneficial or why they are embedded in the way we view ourselves. It is this ability that provides us with normative criteria to define, for example, what actions are moral or what conditions should be rejected. However, again like in Schopenhauer's moral philosophy, this 'why' does not refer back to an *a priori* principle like Kant's categorical imperative or to a notion of 'dignity' based on an *a priori* analysis of the abilities of the rational self, but to empirical observations regarding our responses to suffering and our rejection of situations in which we or others suffer.

Her example of mourning, in the above-cited passage, provides us with an illustration of the manner in which she departs from a Kantian understanding of rationality: even though we may not object to the feeling of grief when a loved one has died, this does not mean that we rationally *choose* to experience grief or that we are free to choose *not* to experience it. Furthermore, it may very well be that in certain cases people actually do *not* want to experience grief but nevertheless are unable to change their feelings. Korsgaard, in other words, reduces her initial notion of *acting in light of reason* to the much weaker *acting for a reason*, arriving at an understanding of rationality that is instrumental in nature – affirming feelings and responses that we *already* have – and comes rather close to Schopenhauer's analysis of the faculty of reason, discussed in Chapter 4.

This means that Schopenhauer's concern with embodiment, especially with corporeal suffering, highlights the problematic nature of attempting to include the negative value we place on pain and suffering within a philosophy that exclusively revolves around reason. In some way or another, we have to refer to our initial negative responses to pain in order to show *why* pain is bad, *why* we reject it and *why* our rejection of this pain is not fundamentally different from the way non-human animals respond to this experience. And even though Schopenhauer does make a distinction between different kinds of pain – thereby accepting the observation that we are able to adopt a reflective distance between our initial negative response to pain and our ideas *about* this pain – the reasons on which we base these evaluations bring us back to our initial negative experiences of pain.

This point can be made more generally: our bodily feelings and responses, Schopenhauer suggests, shape the way we view and experience the world in which we live, ourselves and each other, and our compassionate responses towards other beings provide us with a notion of what we can and cannot do to each other. This is what Korsgaard's struggles with incorporating pain and compassion into an initially Kantian moral philosophy show us: if one wants to do justice to the positive and negative values that these bodily responses provide to certain experiences, one has to let go of the attempt to completely ground a moral philosophy in the faculty of reason and accept the idea that, as corporeal creatures, we always already live in a world filled with values and feelings that influence us, in turn, as thinking creatures.[38]

Injure no one

The fact that we can distil an interesting point from Schopenhauer's observations on pain, compassion and the bodily dimension of our existence does not mean that he is entirely clear about these issues himself, however. In certain passages, it seems, he does not want to make a definite decision regarding the descriptive nature of his moral philosophy and of the norms it provides. This is especially the case regarding his discussion of the normative value of the *incentives* behind our actions and follows from his unclear discussion of the possibility of rational self-control, analysed in Chapter 4.

Claiming that egotism is the strongest 'anti-moral' incentive in human beings – as discussed in Chapter 4 as well – Schopenhauer argues that our criterion for deciding if an action has moral worth is the *complete absence of any egotistic incentives*: an action only has moral worth, in other words, once it is done exclusively and solely for the sake of another.[39] He writes:

> Only insofar as an action has sprung from compassion does it have moral value; and every action resulting from any other motive has

> none. As soon as this compassion is aroused, the weal and woe of another are nearest to my heart in exactly the same way, although not always in the same degree, as otherwise my own are. Hence the difference between him and me is now no longer absolute.[40]

Schopenhauer translates this observation into a principle that can be understood as the 'golden rule' of his moral philosophy: '*Neminem laede, imo omnes, quantum potes, juva*' or 'Injure no one; on the contrary, help everyone as much as you can.'[41]

With this introduction of moral principles that allow us to judge the incentives behind people's actions, Schopenhauer paradoxically provides his descriptive moral philosophy with prescriptive tendencies. In places, he comes close to the idea that we do have some control over our actions. He states, for example: 'Without *principles* firmly held, we should inevitably be at the mercy of anti-moral tendencies when, through external impressions, these tendencies were stirred to emotions. Self-control is the steadfast adherence to and observance of principles, in spite of the motives that act against them.'[42] Even though he claims that the above-mentioned principle is 'by no means the original source or first foundation of morality,'[43] he herewith *does* seem to suggest that human beings can *control* their behaviour by submitting themselves to a principle.

But this latter claim conflicts acutely with Schopenhauer's conclusion that people are completely unfree, enslaved to their innate characters. Indeed, he explicitly states in a paragraph in *On the Basis of Morality* called 'On the Ethical Difference of Characters': 'Is it possible that ethics, in discovering the moral incentive, is also capable of setting it in motion?...Certainly not; the difference of characters is innate and ineradicable. The wicked man is born with his wickedness as much as the serpent is with its poisonous fangs and glands; and he is as little able to change his character as the serpent its fangs.'[44] In his *Essay on the Freedom of the Will* he concludes as well that 'virtues and vices are inborn'.[45]

This means that Schopenhauer's discussion of morality is shaped by a rather uncomfortable tension between, on the one hand, references to moral principles, which in his view not only allow us to make normative distinctions between different forms of behaviour but even to exercise what he calls 'self-control', and on the other hand claims regarding the completely determined nature of human behaviour.

As I have argued in Chapter 4 as well, Schopenhauer's theory on the primacy of Will eventually makes his ideas on human action lean in the direction of the second instead of in the direction of the first understanding of autonomy. And this means that we are forced to conclude that, in the end, rationality plays no constitutive role regarding human behaviour in his moral philosophy. It therefore remains unclear in what way Schopenhauer precisely understands the 'self-control' that is provided by 'firmly held principles': according to his own theory, these principles, after all, follow from the ways in which we *already* act and feel, but cannot determine what we do.

The weakness of compassion

In Chapter 4 we have seen that Schopenhauer argues that 'egoism towers above the world'[46] and is one of the strongest incentives in human beings. More often than not, in other words, this incentive counters the above-described feelings of compassion. Not only does Schopenhauer herewith develop a moral theory that does not tell us what ought to be done but only describes how certain people may respond in certain situations with behaviour that we call moral, he also argues that human beings, most of the time, do not act morally. Furthermore, he observes that moments of compassion are brief in nature, quickly overcome once the subject is 'pulled back' into itself and becomes part of a world defined by the *principium individuationis*:

> ...the illusion of the phenomenon soon ensnares us again, and its motives set the will in motion once more; we cannot tear ourselves free. The allurement of hope, the flattery of the present, the sweetness of pleasures, the well-being that falls to the lot of our person amid the lamentations of a suffering world governed by chance and error, all these draw us back to it, and rivet the bonds anew.[47]

Based on these and other characteristics, many have criticized Schopenhauer's moral philosophy for being weak. In the following, I want to discuss several critical arguments that have been developed against his morality of compassion by Horkheimer, Adorno, Nietzsche and Scheler, and discuss how we may respond to these arguments from a Schopenhauerian point of view.

Inequality

In *Dialectic of Enlightenment* Horkheimer and Adorno criticize Schopenhauer's references to compassion as implicitly affirming the evil of the world. In the above-mentioned chapter on the Marquis De Sade, we find the following analysis of the mechanisms underlying 'pity', the English translation used for the German *Mitleid*:

> By limiting the abolition of injustice to fortuitous love of one's neighbour, pity accepts as unalterable the law of universal estrangement which it would like to alleviate. It is true that the person who shows pity upholds as an individual the claim of the general, that is, the claim to life, against the general in the form of nature and society, which deny it. But the unity with the general as something inward, practiced by such an individual, is shown to be deceptive by his own weakness. It is not the softness but the restrictive nature of pity which makes it questionable – it is always too little.[48]

Pity, Horkheimer and Adorno argue, is based on an implicit affirmation of the idea that the whole in which people suffer, the conditions under which they live, cannot be changed. The only thing we can do, the acceptance of pity suggests, is affirm these conditions while feeling sorry for the suffering that they cause. Adorno and Horkheimer argue against this idea that a situation in which suffering takes place should be rejected *as a whole* and that pity merely 'conforms the rule of inhumanity by the exception it makes'.[49] Instead of references to a mere feeling, Adorno and Horkheimer suggest that a moral philosophy should categorically reject these conditions by embracing a moral theory that, by definition, includes all people and not just those we happen to feel sorry for. Pity, in other words, is never enough.

Adorno makes this same point in his lectures on *Problems of Moral Philosophy*: 'the concept of compassion tacitly maintains and gives its sanction to the negative condition of powerlessness in which the object of our pity finds itself. The idea of compassion contains nothing about changing the circumstances that give rise to the need for it, but instead, as in Schopenhauer, these circumstances are absorbed into the moral doctrine and interpreted as its main foundation.'[50]

Pity and fascism

Horkheimer and Adorno furthermore embed the notion of 'pity' in an analysis of the historical conditions they criticize in *Dialectic of Enlightenment*. They argue that 'bourgeois coldness' – discussed in Chapter 5 – is the 'counterpart' of pity[51] and criticize 'the effusions of philanthropists and the moral complacency of the welfare worker' as 'narcissistic deformations of pity' that are an 'internalized endorsement of the difference between rich and poor'.[52] They even link this idea to the origins of Nazi Germany:

> The fascist masters of the world translated the vilification of pity into that of political respect and the appeal to martial law, in which they were at one with Schopenhauer, the metaphysician of pity. For him the establishment of a humane order was the presumptuous delusion of someone who could hope only for misfortune. The enemies of pity were unwilling to equate humanity with misfortune. For them, the existence of misfortune was a scandal. With their impotent delicacy, they could not bear to see humanity pitied. In desperation their powerlessness switched to the glorification of power, while disowning it in practice whenever it gave them leave.[53]

Not only is the phenomenon of pity not strong enough to hold against those who develop a morality based on coldness and hatred, Adorno and Horkheimer's psychoanalytical reading of this phenomenon suggests, but a world in which humanity is pitied may actually lead to a world in which power and domination are celebrated. They argue that both worlds result from a pathological view of humanity that revolves around a frustrated and neurotic response to feelings of powerlessness. Schopenhauer claims that the world cannot be changed and that human beings are unable to take control over their fate, thereby making 'pity' into an affirmation of not only the suffering that takes place in the world, but also of one's own condition of powerlessness. 'The fascists', in turn, implicitly affirmed this worldview but tried to rebel against the feelings of frustration that it causes by violently celebrating power and a hostility against those who were falsely portrayed as responsible for it.

Horkheimer and Adorno base this analysis of pity on the writings of the Marquis de Sade and Friedrich Nietzsche.[54] In the works of both, pity is portrayed as a sin, they observe, opposing 'the laws of nature'.[55] Indeed, Nietzsche criticizes the phenomenon of *Mitleid* as belonging to the Christian ideology of resentment that he aggressively rejects, writing in *The Gay Science* that 'pity is praised as the virtue of prostitutes'.[56] Furthermore, Nietzsche argues that pity is based on egotism since relieving the sufferer of his pain also relieves the compassionate person of his pity. In *Daybreak*, for example, he observes that 'it is only *this suffering of our own* which we get rid of when we perform deeds of pity'.[57]

But Horkheimer and Adorno do not just follow Nietzsche's critical analysis of *Mitleid*; they also turn against it. The idea that fascist celebrations of power are a neurotic response to the same feelings of powerlessness that spawned Schopenhauer's metaphysics of pity is not just a comment on fascism, but also on Nietzsche's philosophy. Put simplistically: in response to the observation that one has no control over one's fate Schopenhauer rejected the Will and the suffering it causes by affirming feelings of *Mitleid*. Nietzsche, on the other hand, rejected feelings of *Mitleid* and embraced the Will to Power. The philosophies of both follow, in Adorno's view, from rather neurotic attempts to cope with a similar experience. In his lectures on *Problems of Moral Philosophy* Adorno therefore observes: 'Nietzsche's hostility to compassion is a purely abstract negation of Schopenhauer's ethics of compassion, and it was put to the test by the Third Reich and in general by totalitarian states in a way that would have horrified Nietzsche more than anyone.'[58]

We indeed find several passages on pity in Nietzsche's writings that come close to not only Sade's above-mentioned observations on nature but also to social Darwinism. In the seventh paragraph of *The Anti-Christ*, for example, Nietzsche states the following: 'Pity on the whole thwarts the law of evolution, which is the law of selection. It preserves what is ripe for destruction; it defends life's disinherited and condemned; through the abundance of the ill-constituted of all kinds which it retains in life it gives life itself a gloomy and questionable aspect.'[59] Even though Schopenhauer would agree with Nietzsche that *Mitleid* 'thwarts the law of evolution', like Horkheimer and Adorno he would be appalled by the claim that it is therefore wrong: Schopenhauer's moral philosophy is based on a fundamental resistance against the idea that a living being is 'ripe for destruction' because it is not valuable anymore in a world characterized by a struggle for survival.

Pity and compassion

This brings me to an evaluation of the other critical arguments developed by Adorno, Horkheimer and Nietzsche. I agree with these authors that Schopenhauer's moral observations follow from the implicit acceptance of the claim that the world cannot be changed: his philosophy, after all, revolves around the idea that the essence of the universe defines what the world is like and what human beings do. He rejects (Kantian) notions like dignity or rational self-constitution and departs from the idea that human beings can rationally control their own fate. However, it is difficult to argue that *Mitleid* is based on inequality between the one who suffers and the one who experiences *Mitleid*. This observation brings us to the one-sided nature of Lukács' claim that Schopenhauer exclusively affirms egotism, discussed in Chapter 4.

Schopenhauer might agree that, indeed, it is possible that people experience *Mitleid* because they want to feel better about themselves, but he would conclude that the actions triggered by this feeling are not moral in nature. Only the complete absence of egotism makes an act into a *moral* act, according to Schopenhauer. And this means that the only aim of a moral action is preventing or alleviating the suffering of someone else, even though this might bring the compassionate agent him- or herself into trouble. Schopenhauer's insistence on the impulsive, direct and selfless nature of compassion, in other words, goes against the calculating and egotistic agent Nietzsche describes.[60]

It could therefore be argued that Nietzsche's critique, and Adorno and Horkheimer's as well, is aimed at the phenomenon described in German as *Erbarmen* (often used in religious contexts) and not at the phenomenon of *Mitleid*. Whereas *Erbarmen* and 'pity' suggest an inequality between the passivity and dependence of the person in pain and the active and independent position of the compassionate agent, the notions of *Mitleid* and compassion come closer to the radical equality Schopenhauer describes as a result of the removal of the *principium individuationis*. By claiming that the second type of *Mitleid* does not exist and always contains egotistic tendencies, in other words, Nietzsche affirms a view of humanity that is even more cynical than Schopenhauer's and that borders on Sade's above-described nihilism.

This suggests, in other words, that Schopenhauer develops a critique of egotistic forms of *Mitleid* and praises the selflessness of compassion, distinguishing two different responses to suffering. In Chapter 8 I will show that Adorno himself comes close to these ideas on selfless compassion as well.[61]

The negativity of compassion

Nietzsche criticizes Schopenhauer's moral philosophy for another reason. He observes, again in *The Anti-Christ*, that *Mitleid* is a 'depressive and contagious instinct' that 'thwarts those instincts bent on preserving and enhancing the value of life'.[62] A similar point was made by Max Scheler in his 1926 *The Nature of Sympathy*. Scheler argues that Schopenhauer focuses too one-sidedly on suffering and pain since there is no reason for giving compassion with suffering (*Mitleid*) a higher ethical significance over empathy with joy (*Mitfreude*). The only reason why Schopenhauer believes that the first is more fundamental than the other, Scheler argues, is because he concludes that there is more suffering in this world than there is joy.[63]

Scheler goes even further and claims that Schopenhauer's moral philosophy revolves around an *approval* of compassion and therefore an *affirmation* of suffering. In his view, Schopenhauer argues that we are obligated to *cause* suffering in the world because otherwise we would not experience compassion.[64]

This second aspect of Scheler's critique, however, is based on an overly stereotypical reading of Schopenhauer's moral philosophy. Scheler overlooks the fact that Schopenhauer is not concerned with compassion and suffering *in themselves*, but clearly describes how the former phenomenon urges us to eradicate the latter. Put simplistically: a world without suffering is a better world, according to Schopenhauer.[65]

Nietzsche and Scheler's observations *are* correct, however, that Schopenhauer is only concerned with negative experiences like pain and suffering, instead of with positive feelings like joy and pleasure. This is a consequence of his rather unconvincing argument – discussed in Chapter 4 – that whereas we experience pain directly and overwhelmingly, we experience joy merely as an *absence* of pain and suffering.[66] In this respect, his moral philosophy clearly follows from his pessimism.

Conclusion

We have to conclude that Schopenhauer's moral philosophy is quite weak. The most general rule that follows from his observations – 'Injure no one; on the contrary, help everyone as much as you can' – is based on mere descriptions of behaviour that is sparked by the phenomenon of compassion. And since his philosophy revolves around the idea that human beings are, almost by definition, egotistic creatures, the behaviour he refers to as moral is only displayed by *some* people in *some* situations, in his own view.

With reference to Korsgaard, however, I have argued that Schopenhauer's observations on pain, suffering and compassion show us an interesting aspect of the role that these phenomena can play as the normative basis of moral thought. Once we seek to develop a morality that is completely based on *a priori*, rationalistic arguments, Schopenhauer suggests, it is difficult to argue why pain is bad or why our compassionate responses to suffering bodies provide us with normative guidance. In some way or another, we need to include the body in our moral observations instead of cutting it off by focusing on the abstract notion of a purely rational subject.

Again, we herewith arrive at the observation that Schopenhauer's philosophy is too radical and results in unconvincing conclusions, but that it nevertheless contains interesting and valuable ideas, which in this case force us to be critical of those who seek to construct a moral philosophy by solely referring to the faculty of reason.

8
Being a Good Animal

Introduction

The 2012 documentary film *The Act of Killing* revolves around the Indonesian killings of 1965–66, when approximately 500,000 people were accused of holding communist ideals and executed. The documentary follows several men who were part of the death squads that committed these mass murders.[1]

Even though they personally killed hundreds of people, these men are considered heroes. They live in a social and cultural whole in which their crimes are not perceived as crimes: they boast about how many people they killed, how young the girls were that they raped and how efficiently they organized their genocide. One of them is part of a right-wing paramilitary organization that grew out of the death squads and has members that even include ministers of the Indonesian government.

Some of the men justify their crimes by rationalizing counter-arguments away, using observations that remind of the works of the Marquis de Sade, cited in Chapter 7. One of them explains: 'Killing is the worst crime you can do. So the key is to find a way not to feel guilty. It's all about finding the right excuse. For example, if I'm asked to kill someone: if the compensation is right, then of course I'll do it, and from one perspective it's not wrong. That's the perspective we must make ourselves believe. After all, morality is relative.'[2]

When the same person is asked what he thinks of the fact that what he did is defined by the Geneva Conventions as 'war crimes', he gives the following answer:

> I don't necessarily agree with those international laws. When Bush was in power, Guantanamo was right. Saddam Hussein had weapons

> of mass destruction. That was right according to Bush, but now it's wrong. The Geneva Conventions may be today's morality, but tomorrow we'll have the Jakarta Conventions and dump the Geneva conventions. 'War crimes' are defined by the winners. I'm a winner, so I can make my own definition.[3]

Morality, in other words, constantly changes and one can use this observation as an argument for the claim that executing people may be the right thing to do. His ability to reflect upon history, culture and his place in the world, to rationally analyse the nature of his own actions, enables this person to defend the idea that genocide, rape and torture are permitted, at least for him.[4]

The director of *The Act of Killing*, Joshua Oppenheimer, asks the men to re-enact what they did during the killings, which results in one of the most powerful scenes of the documentary. One of them – Anwar – personally killed approximately thousand people by strangling them with a thin metal wire. He re-enacts this at the same rooftop he used for his executions, explaining how the method he used was efficient as well as clean. During the re-enactment of an interrogation, however, Anwar plays the role of a victim: he is blindfolded and pretends to be tortured. After doing this for a while, he suddenly cannot continue: he begins to realize what he actually did and how much the people he tortured suffered. He is unable to really explain his feelings, but his body simply stops working: he cannot move or talk anymore and almost faints.

When they return to the rooftop where he strangled his victims, Anwar says: 'This is where we tortured and killed the people we captured. I know it was wrong but I had to do it. Why did I have to kill them? I had to kill.... My conscience told me they had to be killed.' Holding up a metal wire and a jute bag, he proceeds: 'This is... this is one of the easiest ways to take a human life. And this... this was used to take away the human beings we killed. Because without this maybe people would know.'[5]

When he is recounting this, Anwar starts to gag violently, which goes on for several minutes. Starting to realize how horrible his deeds were and how much suffering he has caused, he can do nothing else than refer to the efficiency of the tools he used and cling vaguely to the idea that his conscience told him to kill and torture. Living in a cultural and social whole that tells him that his actions were not crimes but heroic deeds, his body literally confronts his crumbling self with the sickening nature of what he did, loathing the barbarity of his crimes.

Life does not live

In this chapter I will discuss Adorno's moral philosophy and develop an interpretation of his references to the addendum in a moral context. In my interpretation of this latter notion, several of the above-discussed aspects of *The Act of Killing* return.

The attempt to base a moral philosophy on Adorno's works is acutely undermined by the radical negativity of his observations. Citing the Austrian 19th century author Ferdinand Kürnberger's statement that 'life does not live'[6] and adding that 'wrong life cannot be lived rightly',[7] Adorno makes it impossible to refer to a notion of 'the good life' or even of 'living' itself. The falseness of a social whole in which we are not able to discern morally right from morally wrong actions, he suggests, eventually corrodes the possibility of autonomous self-constitution, making it impossible to fully develop a healthy self, embedded in a world it trusts. Instead, this self is only trying to survive and does not have the ability to fully grasp its situation. In his essay on Beckett's *Endgame*, Adorno therefore concludes that 'there has been no life other than the wrong life.'[8]

In his essay 'Cultural Criticism and Society' he puts this problem famously into words as follows: 'Cultural criticism finds itself faced with the final stage of the dialectic of culture and barbarism. To write poetry after Auschwitz is barbaric. And this corrodes even the knowledge of why it has become impossible to write poetry today.'[9] We live in a world in which there are no values to cling to anymore and in which we, furthermore, are not even able to argue *why* this situation is wrong, he argues.

A result of these observations is that Adorno rejects the idea that we can find normatively binding values and norms within the culture and society in which we live. In his sixteenth lecture on *Problems of Moral Philosophy* he therefore criticizes the Hegelian notion of 'ethical life', which revolves around 'responsibility' towards others embedded in a social whole. He argues that this approach to ethics does not do justice to the idea that 'there is no good life in the bad one', that embedding individuals in a false social whole only *affirms* the state of the world instead of *criticizing* it:[10] 'what the ethics of responsibility amounts to is that existing reality – or what Hegel calls the way of the world [*der Weltlauf*], which he defends against the vanity of protesting interiority – is always in the right over against the human subject.'[11]

Another problem with basing a moral philosophy on Adorno's works is that the critical, paradoxical and essayistic style of his writings refuses to be translated into a systematic and robust theory. To a certain extent, it seems, any attempt to base a moral philosophy on his works is doomed to fail since these works themselves resist this. Although Bernstein rightly notes in the first sentence of his influential book on Adorno's ethics that 'no readings of the works of T. W. Adorno can fail to be struck by the ethical intensity of his writing, sentence by sentence, word by word',[12] this 'ethical intensity' shines *through the lines* of his writing and, once conceptualized or theorized, loses that which Adorno values.

Nevertheless, in the following I want to develop the argument that it is possible to distil a moral theory from Adorno's fragmented references to self-critique, compassion, the addendum, pain and suffering. Since Adorno, like Schopenhauer, does this mainly against the background of Kant's *Critique of Practical Reason*, I will begin my discussion of his moral theory with his reading of Kant.

Kant's practical philosophy

Criticizing Kant

Most of Schopenhauer's critique of the formalism of Kant's categorical imperative returns in Adorno's works – embedded, however, in a critical social theory. Adorno claims, for example, that the Kantian idea of submitting oneself to an unconditional imperative results in a submission to social norms and values that formed one as a child. In his lectures on *Problems of Moral Philosophy* he refers to the human 'compulsion' to turn to a moral law, echoing Schopenhauer's claim that Kant defends a disguised theological morality that triggers feelings of approval and fear. In *Dialectic of Enlightenment* Schopenhauer's ideas even return quite literally in the claim that Kant tried to 'transform the divine law into an autonomous principle'.[13] Adorno infuses Schopenhauer's critique with psychoanalytic insights:[14]

> Psychoanalysis in its strict form has shown that these compulsive mechanisms that we are subject to are phylogenetic, that is to say, they are internalisations of actual power, internalisations of dominant social norms. These norms are transmitted to us through the family and we generally appropriate them by identifying with father figures.[15]

Following his critical analysis of instrumental rationality, discussed in Chapters 5 and 6, Adorno furthermore describes the categorical imperative as 'nothing but the principle for achieving the domination of nature, raised to a norm, elevated into an absolute',[16] and claims that 'Kantian morality is at root nothing other than domination'.[17]

Adorno also criticizes the formalism of Kant's morality by attacking its focus on *intentions*. Moral philosophy, he herewith suggests, should always include the specific historical situation in which moral problems arise and do this by taking into account every aspect of this empirical situation. Referring to Henrik Ibsen's play *The Wild Duck*, he therefore argues that one should always take the *consequences* of one's actions into account.[18] *The Wild Duck* provides us, in his reading, with an example of a man who 'becomes immoral by defending the moral law – or, ... by defending the ethical commandments in their purity. To be specific, he brings about the destruction of ... the most valuable human being of the entire group', illustrating the idea that 'a pure moral demand can by virtue of its own purity be transformed into evil'.[19]

In the excursus on Sade, this aspect of Kant's emphasis on rationality is criticized as follows: 'Sade demonstrated empirically what Kant grounded transcendentally: the affinity between knowledge and planning which has set its stamp of inescapable functionality on a bourgeois existence rationalized even in its breathing spaces'.[20]

This critique of the rationalization of every aspect of existence is related to Adorno's claim, discussed in Chapter 6, that Kant's moral philosophy 'excludes all desires and impulses'.[21] Kant's emphasis on the purity of rational self-constitution, Adorno argues repeatedly, reflects a hostility towards bodily feelings and needs, embodying the schism between mind and body that he links to the rise of the enlightened self (I quoted an exemplary passage from Kant's *Groundwork of the Metaphysics of Morals* in my analysis of Korsgaard's understanding of compassion and pain in Chapter 7).

Schopenhauer's observation that 'in the storm and stress of life' one never turns to 'the a priori building of houses of cards' also returns in an example Adorno develops, concerning a refugee coming to one's door and asking for shelter: 'if reason makes its entrance at this point then reason itself becomes irrational.'[22] Kant's notion of the categorical imperative, Adorno concludes, is based on the overly abstract idea of an 'absolute independence from all existing beings', which forces the subject to overlook the specifics of the situations it find itself in, as Ibsen's above-mentioned play shows us, in his view.[23] Whereas Adorno criticizes Hegelian ethics, in other words, for embedding the subject too deeply in a false social whole, he argues that Kant's philosophy is equally unrealistic because it completely pulls this subject out of this whole and looks at it from a purely rational, abstract point of view.

Defending Kant

Like Schopenhauer, Adorno's Kant-critique is based on a rather stereotypical and unfavourable interpretation of Kant. Again, it could be argued that Kant does not so much reject actions based on desires or inclinations, but that he claims that we cannot speak of *moral* actions once we act on desires or inclinations. Kant, in other words, formulates a highly critical notion of morality aimed at realizing the *ability* we have as rational and reflective creatures instead of merely accepting what he would regard as the too relativistic idea that we should act on our inclinations.[24]

Furthermore, Adorno seems to suggest, like Schopenhauer, that Kant argues that the subject is only free once it conforms its will to a rational law. A more subtle reading of Kant, however, allows one to claim that the reflective subject can be free because it pulls itself out of a deterministic world defined by a chain of cause and effect *without* claiming that this subject has to submit itself to a rational law. Kant makes a difference, in other words, between complete determinism on the one hand and on the other both the freedom to not follow one's bodily inclinations *and* the freedom attained by constituting oneself as a moral and autonomous creature.[25] This means that Adorno forces an either/or of complete determinism *or* complete rational self-constitution on Kant's philosophy that overlooks a more subtle middle-ground.

Like Schopenhauer, however, I believe that Adorno is mainly criticizing that which Kant's moral philosophy represents, in his view: a submission to laws – which Adorno understands as social in nature – that overlooks the idea that the subject is always an embodied subject, embedded in a social and cultural world. As we will see in the following, Adorno defends a more pragmatic moral philosophy that takes our specific responses in historically shaped situations into account instead of one that constructs an abstract ideal based on the theoretical abilities of a purely rational subject.[26]

Self-critique and the moral addendum

We have now seen that Adorno both rejects values embedded in a social community and rational self-constitution as possible normative grounds of a moral philosophy. He therefore turns to a specific interpretation of his concept of the addendum to provide his moral thought with a spark of normativity.

In the following I will develop an interpretation of his references to this moral addendum by looking at the nature of pain and suffering. I will structure the arguments leading up to this interpretation similarly to the analysis developed in Chapter 6: first I will discuss Adorno's positive discussion of rationality and self-reflection, then his ideas on the moral addendum. Using a similar structure allows me to show that Adorno's claim that the rational self needs to be infused with a non-rational element in order to act, discussed in Chapter 6, is similar to his idea that the addendum forms the normative basis of his philosophy. Based on this observation, I will argue that Adorno implies that the phenomenon that sets the subject in motion is at the same time the normative basis of his moral thought, which means that the *descriptive* aspects of Adorno's ideas on action and rationality are entwined with, and in places even similar to its *normative* elements.

Self-critique

An important part of Adorno's moral philosophy revolves around the critical potential of rational reflection, which I partly discussed in Chapter 6. Whereas Adorno criticizes certain aspects of Kant's moral philosophy, his defence of rational self-critique revolves around an affirmation of other aspects of Kant's thought. In his lectures on *Problems of Moral Philosophy*, for example, we find the following defence of Kant against Hegel's ethics: 'Kant's principle of universality elevates his ethics above every determinate configuration of the world that confronts it, above society and existing conditions, and it also makes him more critical of limited and finite moral categories.'[27]

This affirmation of a critical attitude towards 'limited and finite moral categories' provides Adorno with an alternative to Schopenhauer's morality of compassion. In Chapter 7 we have seen that he criticizes compassion for implicitly affirming the conditions under which people suffer by claiming that we cannot change them. Compassion constitutes inequality between people, he argues, and affirms the wrongness of the status quo. Furthermore, Adorno holds the Kantian concern that feelings of compassion are fleeting and make the basis of moral thought contingent and unreliable. By holding on to the ideas of critique and rational reflection Adorno seeks to overcome these limitations.

In his lectures Adorno returns again and again to this positive aspect of Kant's philosophy: 'We need to hold fast to moral norms, to self-criticism, to the question of right and wrong, and at the same time to a sense of the fallibility of the authority that has the confidence to undertake such self-criticism.'[28] This reference to fallibility brings us to one of the key moments of Adorno's moral philosophy: the idea that one should never imprison oneself within the walls of one's own thought and proclaim that one is always right. In his last lecture on *Problems of Moral Philosophy* we find a long passage that contains one of the most explicit and clear formulations of Adorno's understanding of the 'right life':

> I would say that the element of self-reflection has today become the true heir to what used to be called moral categories. This means that if today we can at all say that subjectively there is something like a threshold, a distinction between a right life and a wrong one, we are likely to find it soonest in asking whether a person is just hitting out blindly at other people – while claiming that the group to which he belongs is the only positive one, and other groups should be negated – or whether by reflecting on our own limitations we can learn to do justice to those who are different, and to realize that true injustice is always to be found at the precise point where you put yourself in the right and other people in the wrong. Hence to abstain from self-assertiveness ... seems to me to be the crucial thing to ask from individuals today. In other words, if you were to press me to follow the example of the Ancients and make a list of the cardinal virtues, I would probably respond cryptically by saying that I could think of nothing except for modesty. Or to put it another way, we must have a conscience, but may not insist on our own conscience.[29]

Rational critique does not affirm or embrace the social whole in which we find ourselves, in Adorno's view, but hovers above it and criticizes it with all its force.[30] Furthermore, it forces us to think about our responses and feelings and to elevate ourselves to a level from which we are able to discern the limitations of, for example, a moral concept like compassion and of our ideas in general.

The moral addendum

It is important to notice that Adorno only praises the *critical* and *analytical* capacities of the faculty of reason, rejecting the idea that, from a purely rational point of view, *a priori* norms can be constructed that provide us with guiding, normative criteria. Adorno therefore returns to his understanding of the addendum, of which he develops a specific interpretation in the context of morality. I want to argue in the following that this interpretation makes his moral philosophy more similar to Schopenhauer's than he himself suggested.

As in the context of action, in which Adorno refers to 'the twitching of the hand', he contrasts the moral addendum with a rational subject that suppresses everything somatic. In *Against Epistemology*, briefly discussed in Chapter 2, he indeed links both realms – that of freedom and that of morality – by referring as follows to the 'bit of nature' that cannot be usurped by the notion of a 'pure consciousness': 'the material element simply cannot be rooted out of it. Bordering on physical pain and organic desire, it is a bit of nature which cannot be reduced to subjectivity.'[31]

In the context of his moral philosophy, Adorno defines the addendum as the experience of compassion with this 'physical pain', by which he mainly refers to the horrors of Auschwitz. Adorno writes about 'a bodily sensation of the moral addendum – bodily, because it is now the practical abhorrence of the unbearable physical agony to which individuals are exposed even with individuality about to vanish as a form of mental reflection'.[32] And in another passage he refers to the addendum in this context as a 'remainder': 'moral action cannot be wholly translated into its theoretical determinants without remainder.'[33] In one of his most-quoted passages on morality he refers to a similar 'impulse', this time not using the concept 'addendum':

> It is not in their nauseating parody, sexual repression, that moral questions are succinctly posed: it is in lines such as: No man should be tortured; there should be no concentration camps – while all of this continues in Asia and Africa and is repressed merely because, as ever, the humanity of civilisation is inhumane toward the people it shamelessly brands as uncivilized. ... The lines are true as an impulse, as a reaction to the news that torture is going on somewhere. They must not be rationalized; as an abstract principle they would fall promptly into the bad infinities of derivation and validity. ... The impulse – naked physical fear, and the sense of solidarity with what Brecht called 'tormentable bodies' – is immanent in moral conduct and would be denied in attempts at ruthless rationalization.[34]

In the context of morality, in other words, the addendum should be understood as a corporeal shock of compassion with suffering beings, a shock about which Adorno explicitly claims that it cannot and should not be rationalized, and which he not only embeds in the context of Auschwitz but also links to 'Asia' and 'Africa'.

In Chapter 6 we have seen that several of Schopenhauer's ideas on the inability of the Kantian subject to act return in Adorno's analysis of the addendum. Now another important theme within Schopenhauer's philosophy returns: compassion with bodily suffering. Again – like 'the twitching of the hand' – Adorno refers to this addendum as a frail and almost completely overshadowed bodily feeling. In his own words: as 'a last epistemological quiver of the somatic element, before that element is totally expelled'.[35] And again, these references add a naturalistic dimension to Adorno's thought; he places them almost in direct opposition to the mediating influences of culture: 'suffering is objectivity that weighs upon the subject.'[36]

In his fifteenth lecture on metaphysics we find perhaps Adorno's most explicit claim regarding the moral dimension of corporeality:

> If I say to you that the true basis of morality is to be found in bodily feeling, in identification with unbearable pain, I am showing you from a different side something which I earlier tried to indicate in a far more abstract form. It is that morality, that which can be called moral, i.e. the demand for right living, lives on in openly materialist motifs. The metaphysical principle of the injunction that 'Thou shalt not inflict pain' – and this injunction is a metaphysical principle pointing beyond mere facticity – can find its justification only in the recourse to material reality, to corporeal, physical reality, and not to its opposite pole, the pure idea. Metaphysics, I say, has slipped into material existence. Precisely this transition of metaphysical questions and, if I might state it so grandly, of metaphysics itself to the stratum of the material, is what is repressed by the conniving consciousness, the official yes-saying of whatever ilk. As a child, I believe, one still knows something about this stratum – with the dim knowledge people have of such things. It is the zone which later materialized literally in the concentration camps; as a child one had an inkling of it in subliminal experiences – as when the dog-catcher's van drove by, or suchlike things: one knew that that was the most important thing of all, that was what really mattered, the zone of the carcass and the knacker.[37]

In the 'Meditations on Metaphysics' in *Negative Dialectics*, Adorno refers again to the haunting image of the dog-catcher's van: 'A child, fond of an innkeeper named Adam, watched him club the rats pouring out of holes in the courtyard; it was in his image that the child made its own image of the first man. That this has been forgotten, that we no longer know what we used to feel before the dogcatcher's van, is both the triumph of culture and its failure.'[38]

Adorno here develops a radical judgement of the culture in which we live and the consciousness it has constituted: both stimulate the ability to overcome our compassion for vulnerable creatures – human and non-human – and thereby enhance the capacity to hurt others or to look away when others are hurt. Adorno explicitly links this attitude of coldness – discussed in Chapter 4 – to the ability to hurt animals and praises Schopenhauer in this context for emphasizing the blindness of Kant's categorical imperative to animal suffering by referring 'to the weak point in the transition from subjective reason concerned with self-preservation to the supreme moral principle, which has no room for animals and our treatment of animals'.[39]

Adorno and Schopenhauer on compassion

It is the shocking nature of our rejection of suffering that forms the normative basis of Adorno's moral philosophy, I want to argue in the following, which means that whereas he claims that the addendum is needed to provide the rational subject with spontaneity, with a drive that enables it to act, he also argues that this addendum presents the subject with a moral norm.[40] Our compassionate responses to suffering creatures, Adorno suggests, demand something from us, force us to respond morally. In the aphorism 'People are looking at you', a reference to Paul Eipper's book 'Animals are looking at you' (*Tiere siehen dich an*[41]), Adorno makes this point as follows, again describing animal-cruelty:

> The possibility of pogroms is decided in the moment when the gaze of a fatally-wounded animal falls on a human being. The defiance with which he repels this gaze – 'after all, it's only an animal' – reappears irresistibly in cruelties done to human beings, the perpetrators having again and again to reassure themselves that it is 'only an animal', because they could never fully believe this even of animals.[42]

The observation that Adorno argues that these perpetrators had to assure themselves that 'it is only an animal' and that he refers to the moral addendum as a 'last quivering remainder' left to the commodified subject, suggest that the nature of pain and the experience of compassion with suffering beings makes it difficult to completely rationalize these phenomena away or quieten them down by embedding them in a culture that is wrong. It is this same quality that enables these phenomena, in Adorno's view, to form the normative basis of moral thought.

This means that even though, as we have seen in Chapter 7, Adorno criticizes moralities of compassion for implicitly affirming injustice, his own references to compassion, pain, suffering and cruelty to animals actually bring him very close to Schopenhauer's moral observations. We have seen that the golden rule that follows from Schopenhauer's descriptive references to feelings of compassion goes as follows: *Neminem laede, imo omnes, quantum potes, juva* or 'Injure no one; on the contrary, help everyone as much as you can'.[43] In the passage cited above, Adorno bases a similar norm on his descriptions of the moral addendum: 'Thou shalt not inflict pain'.[44]

I have argued in Chapter 7 that Schopenhauer's references to compassion contain a critique of a type of *Mitleid* that is based on egotism: only a complete absence of selfish motives constitutes a moral act, in his view. A similar affirmation of selfless acts of compassion now returns in Adorno's moral philosophy. He develops a radical understanding of compassion that not only follows from the idea that every bodily being (human and non-human) is equally vulnerable to pain, but that he also contrasts with culture, thought and philosophy. Whereas Schopenhauer, in other words, criticizes feelings of compassion that are mediated by the *principium individuationis* and egotism, Adorno rejects compassion that is mediated by coldness and by a culture defined by a pathological drive to self-preservation.[45]

Both authors hereby refuse to embed our bodily responses to beings that are in pain in a theory that *provides* these phenomena with normativity. Instead, they suggest that pain *itself* carries an intrinsically negative normativity, an observation that I have discussed in Chapter 7 with reference to Korsgaard.[46] As we have seen in Chapter 7, Volker Spierling characterizes Schopenhauer's moral philosophy in this context as follows:

> Die existentiellen Leiderfahrungen in den primären Anschauungen lassen sich mit sekundären Begriffen *nur bei geschlossenen Augen* wegphilosophieren. Schopenhauer versucht, philosophischen Rechtfertigungen des Leids einen Riegel vorzuschieben. Er stellt der Philosophie den Schmerz des Leibes in den Weg.[47]

In a similar passage in *Negative Dialectics* Adorno describes the contrast between pain and 'identitarian philosophy' as follows:

> The smallest trace of senseless suffering in the empirical world belies all the identitarian philosophy that would talk us out of that suffering:

> 'While there is a beggar, there is a myth,' as Benjamin put it. This is why the philosophy of identity of the mythological form of thought. The physical moment tells our knowledge that suffering ought not to be, that things should be different. 'Woe speaks: "Go."'[48]

Our compassion with suffering others tells us that their pain should not be: pain bears an intrinsic negativity, Adorno claims, and we only have to contrast it with philosophies that seek to justify the existence of suffering to unmask these forms of thought as empty and abstract.[49] In fact, Adorno argues, this feeling of compassion is the only moral response left: the moment we start to reflect on this bodily shock of abhorrence at the perception of suffering people or embed it in a fully-fledged moral theory, we are already distancing ourselves from its initially shocking nature, rationalizing it and thereby making it part of a wrong whole. Adorno observes: 'Practice is when it hurts, when it really hurts.'[50]

This insistence that the addendum cannot and should not be rationalized makes Adorno's moral philosophy both more radical and more problematic than Schopenhauer's. Whereas the latter at least makes it possible to develop a theory about the exact nature of compassion, Adorno refers rather vaguely to a bodily shock that loses its power the moment we begin to reflect on it. Like 'the twitching of the hand' – the example Adorno develops in the context of action, discussed in Chapter 6 – he thereby not only seems to make it impossible, like Schopenhauer, to distinguish the descriptive from the normative, fact from value, but even to philosophically analyse these facts.

Commentators are therefore undecided about the extent to which the addendum is or can be rationalized, in Adorno's view. Some stress the direct and unmediated nature of the addendum. Others argue that Adorno's emphasis on cultural mediation implies that the addendum is always a product of historical and cultural concepts and needs to be reflected upon in order for it to play a role in moral thought.[51] The vague and ungraspable aura that surrounds Adorno's own sparse references to the addendum does not provide us with much more clarity about these issues.

Pain

The dominance of pain

In the following I want to develop an interpretation of these problematic aspects of Adorno's moral philosophy by discussing three analyses of the suffering body: Elaine Scarry's *The Body in Pain*, Jean Améry's *At the Mind's Limits: Contemplations by a Survivor on Auschwitz and its Realities*, and Arne Johan Vetlesen's *A Philosophy of Pain*. In these works we find descriptions of pain that focus on the extreme and rather unique nature of its experience and thereby provide us with a way to interpret Adorno's references to the moral addendum.

In the first chapter of *The Body in Pain* Scarry describes eight characteristics of pain, relying on reports from victims of torture and medical analyses of what happens to a body when it undergoes torture. Of these characteristics, the first, fifth, sixth and seventh are relevant in light of Adorno's references to the addendum and to 'tormentable bodies'. To illustrate this point, I want to quote a large part of Scarry's analysis:

> The first, the most essential, aspect of pain is its sheer aversiveness. While other sensations have content that may be positive, neutral, or negative, the very content of pain is itself negation. If to the person in pain it does not feel averse, and if it does not in turn elicit in that person aversive feelings toward it, it is not in either philosophical discussions or psychological definitions of it called pain. Pain is a pure physical experience of negation, and immediate sensory rendering of 'against,' of something being against one, and of something one must be against. Even though it occurs within oneself, it is at once identified as 'not oneself,' 'not me,' as something so alien that it must be gotten rid of....
>
> A fifth dimension of physical pain is its ability to destroy language, the power of verbal objectification, a major source of our self-extension.... Before destroying language, it first monopolizes language, becomes its only subject: complaint...becomes the exclusive mode of speech. Eventually the pain so deepens that the coherence of complaint is displayed by the sounds anterior to language....
>
> A sixth element of physical pain, one that overlaps but is not quite coterminous with the previous element, is its obliteration of the contents of consciousness. Pain annihilates not only the objects of complex thought and emotion but also the objects of the most elemental acts of perception.
>
> A seventh aspect of pain...is its totality. Pain begins by being 'not oneself' and ends by having eliminated all that is 'not itself.' At first occurring only as an appalling but limited internal fact, it eventually occupies the entire body and spills out into the realm beyond the body, takes over all that is inside and outside, makes the two obscenely indistinguishable, and systematically destroys anything

> like language or world extension that is alien to itself and threatening to its claims.[52]

These characterizations come very close to those developed by Jean Améry, an Austrian essayist who survived the concentration camps of Auschwitz, Buchenwald and Bergen-Belsen.[53] In 'Torture', one of the chapters in *At the Mind's Limits*, Améry describes his experiences in the Belgian Gestapo center in Fort Breendonk, where he was imprisoned for being part of the underground resistance. The Gestapo tortured Améry, trying to extract information from him. As follows Améry describes the way in which extreme pain reduces one to one's body, transforming one 'thoroughly into flesh':[54]

> Whoever is overcome by pain through torture experiences his body as never before. In self-negation, his flesh becomes total reality. Partially, torture is one of those life experiences that in a milder form present themselves also to the consciousness of the patient who is awaiting help, and the popular saying according to which we feel well as long as we do not feel our body does indeed express an undeniable truth. But only in torture does the transformation of the person into flesh become complete. Frail in the face of violence, yelling out in pain, awaiting no help, capable of no resistance, the tortured person is only a body, and nothing else beside that.[55]

Both Améry and Scarry argue that the extreme pain that victims of torture undergo robs them of their individuality and reduces them to a suffering body; to screaming flesh. Both furthermore claim that the subject ceases to exist in this state: not only is it unable to reflect on this situation, to rationalize it or to grasp it in a meaningful way, it is also unable to put it into words and to tell what such an experience is like. 'If someone wanted to impart this physical pain', Valéry writes, 'he would be forced to inflict it and thereby become a torturer himself'.[56]

Similar observations return in Arne Johan Vetlesen's *A Philosophy of Pain*. With the following statement Vetlesen criticizes Jean-Paul Sartre's idea that the truly free individual can *choose* to reject or accept pain:

> [P]ain is not just any state or feeling. [... P]ain is characterized by its lack of distance, by its directness: my pain fills me, marks me, with an immediacy and permeability that are in stark contrast to Sartre's analysis.... Pain does something to us, changes and transforms us, and the reality of this aspect of experiencing pain – that pain is an experience

> in the strict sense that strikes and shakes us and causes everything to be altered – is lost in Sartre's insistence on freedom and choice.[57]

Vetlesen's critique reminds one of Adorno's dismissal of Sartre's claim that even the victims of Auschwitz could *choose* to accept or reject their situation, which I mentioned in the conclusion to Chapter 7. Physical pain destroys this illusion, corrodes the idea of an autonomous subject and pulls the suffering individual into a materiality in which the idea of accepting or rejecting this pain ceases to exist. As Vetlesen observes: 'pain heaves the ego down from the pedestal.'[58]

The ungraspability of pain

An important consequence of these analyses of pain is that this experience cannot be conceptualized or put into language. Scarry writes in *The Body in Pain*:

> moving through the human interior, one at last reached physical pain, for physical pain – unlike any other state of consciousness – has no referential content. It is not of or for anything. It is precisely because it takes no object that it, more than any other phenomenon, resists objectification in language.[59]

In other words: extreme pain cannot be grasped, understood, sensed like we sense objects around us. Furthermore, extreme pain cannot be controlled; it cannot be structured or organized rationally. In fact, as Améry, Scarry and Vetlesen show, pain corrodes the ability to reason, to form judgements, to talk or to keep a sense of one's self as a unified whole.

I want to argue that these characteristics echo through Adorno's moral philosophy. According to this reading one cannot argue *why* pain is wrong because one has lost the ability to argue or to reflect *at all* if one experiences the kinds of suffering that Adorno refers to. Furthermore, the situations in which these kinds of suffering take place are so overwhelmingly negative and so distorting at a rather primitive 'level' of experience that the difference disappears between oneself as a reflective individual and other individuals and is replaced by a categorical physical rejection of the situation *as a whole*.

Adorno, in other words, refers to a kind of suffering – being placed in a concentration camp, undergoing torture, murder, medical experimentation, extreme famine and extreme coldness – that is so all-engulfing and so 'totalizing', that it reduces the people that undergo this suffering to their bodies, to the pain they experience, drowning out the ability to reason and to reflect. In *At the Mind's Limits* Jean Améry described this kind of suffering as follows by referring to the concept of the 'musselman':

> The so-called musselman, as the camp language termed the prisoner who was giving up and was given up by his comrades, no longer had room in his consciousness for the contrasts good or bad, noble or base, intellectual or unintellectual. He was a staggering corpse, a bundle or physical functions in its last convulsions.[60]

Adorno's references to the moral addendum, I want to argue, can be understood as revolving around physical compassion with people living in this 'middle ground', 'inhabited by living skeletons and putrefying bodies, victims unable to take their own lives';[61] in a 'place of carrion, stench and putrefaction' in which they 'vegetate between life and death'.[62]

The specificity of pain

This interpretation introduces an important difference between Schopenhauer and Adorno's observations on morality. Whereas Schopenhauer refers to compassion as following from the essential nature of the universe – Will – and thereby as a universal human capacity, Adorno links the experience of solidarity with suffering beings to a specific, historical situation: Nazi Germany and the construction of the death camps.[63] As he observes in *Aesthetic Theory*: 'suffering conceptualized remains mute and inconsequential, as is obvious in post-Hitler Germany.'[64]

Even though Adorno's descriptions of compassion and suffering contain naturalistic tendencies, referring to compassion with animals and bodily shock moments that are devoid of rationality, they do, in other words, arise from a specific historical situation in which a specific kind of suffering takes place.

Following the analyses developed by Améry, Scarry and Vetlesen, which tell us that extreme kinds of pain drown out the subject's ability to reason or even to reflect, I want to argue that Adorno's insistence that the addendum cannot and should not be rationalized implies that he refers here specifically to extreme kinds of pain, to torture and genocide, to the suffering that took place in the concentration camps. In other words: even though the addendum may not be rationalized and, at places, appears to be an almost causal bodily response, this does not mean that it is not historical in nature or aimed at specific phenomena.

This interpretation is substantiated by the observation, discussed in Chapter 6, that Adorno's references to bodily impulses do not revolve around *completely* unmediated aspects of nature: he does not refer to instincts but to drives, to bodily responses that are entwined with and influenced by specific, historically constituted situations, following from psychoanalytic insights regarding the entwinement of body and mind.[65]

As an example that illustrates this interpretation, I want to refer to Anwar, one of the members of the Indonesian death squads shown in the above-discussed *The Act of Killing*. Living in a social and cultural whole in which his deeds are praised, claiming that his conscience told him to execute innocent people, Anwar is unable to really distinguish right from wrong. At a deeply repressed level, however, he suspects or even realizes that his deeds were evil and that he cannot make them right by talking about the relative nature or morality or by rationalizing counter-arguments away. To a certain extent, his ego shields him off from his feelings of guilt, but his body loathes his actions and expresses that which he cannot rationally, conceptually or even consciously reach or grasp.

This corporeal response, however, is not completely instinctive in nature, which illustrates my interpretation of Adorno's references to the moral addendum: it is entwined with Anwar's ideas, his memories, and his existences as a person with a specific history living in a specific context. But it also has a deeply materialistic undertone, being a bodily response to something that his mind cannot cope with.

The universality of pain

Another important aspect of my interpretation rests on the idea that the kind of suffering Adorno refers to drowns out the ability to reflect and conceptualize not only 'in' the victims themselves but also in those confronted with their suffering; *even* – and this is the most extreme aspect of this analysis – *in those who try to say anything on a philosophical level about this suffering*. It could be argued, after all, that victims of extreme torture may not be able to form normative judgements about their situation, but that people who are not in their situation *are* capable of doing this. Adorno *also* rejects the latter claim according to my interpretation. In his lectures on *Metaphysics* we find a passage that substantiates this idea:

> It might be said that in view of what we have experienced – and let me say that it is also experienced by those on whom it was not directly perpetrated – there can be no one, whose organ of experience

> has not entirely atrophied, for whom the world *after* Auschwitz, that is, the world in which Auschwitz was possible, is the same world as it was before.... I would say, therefore, that these experiences have a compelling universality.[66]

This does not mean that Adorno, in my view, suggests that the philosopher who tries to say something about a suffering victim is in the same situation as that victim, but that the specific historical, social and political context that he describes, a context in which the suffering of victims could take place on such an enormous and industrially organized scale and was almost collectively rationalized away or even presented as necessary, is the same false context in which the philosopher tries to say something about this suffering.

A new categorical imperative

Auschwitz never again

In *Negative Dialectics* Adorno bases a 'new categorical imperative' on the moral addendum:

> A new categorical imperative has been imposed by Hitler upon unfree mankind: to arrange their thoughts and actions so that Auschwitz will not repeat itself, so that nothing similar will happen. When we want to find reasons for it, this imperative is as refractory as the given one of Kant was once upon a time. Dealing discursively with it would be an outrage, for the new imperative gives us a bodily sensation of the moral addendum – bodily, because it is now the practical abhorrence of the unbearable physical agony to which individuals are exposed even with individuality about to vanish as a form of mental reflection. It is in this unvarnished materialistic motive only that morality survives.[67]

The specific historical situation in which Adorno seeks to construct his moral philosophy – 'Hitler Germany' – provides him with a normative basis – a corporeal experience – that results in a categorical rejection of that same situation. Again, he explicitly argues that this imperative is not rational or conceptual in nature, but nevertheless emphasizes its absolute nature:

> It is impossible to found this imperative on logic – it has that in common with the Kantian imperative. When Kant states that his

> own imperative is simply given, that assertion doubtless contains all kinds of grimly authoritarian and irrationalist elements, but also ... an awareness that the sphere of right action does not coincide with mere rationality, that it has an 'addendum'. I believe that an attempt to state as a general law why Auschwitz or the atom bomb or all those things which belong together here should not be repeated would have something utterly feeble about it because it would transfer into the sphere of rationality, which is ultimately the secondary sphere of mind, the right to a jurisdiction which it can only usurp.[68]

In a rather Schopenhauerian manner Adorno here describes the faculty of reason as a secondary function and as something 'added' to our existence. Our bodies tell us that suffering is wrong ('Woe speaks: "Go"', as he quotes Nietzsche's *Zarathustra's Rundgesang*), and this rejection of violence, hatred, pain and suffering functions as a normative basis of moral thought.

This means that the 'why' behind the wrongness of pain and suffering is not rational or based on *a priori* constructed principles. But it does not mean that rationality does not play an important role in Adorno's moral philosophy. This brings us back to his references to modesty and self-critique, which have been discussed above. If feelings of abhorrence that we experience when we are confronted with the sufferings of other people tell us that the whole in which we live is wrong, a process of self-critique may be set in motion, Adorno suggests, which forces us to reflect on our ideas and our tendencies but also on the culture in which we live.

I want to argue that these observations eventually result in what I want to characterize as a moral *attitude* towards the world in which rationality *does* play an important role, unlike in Schopenhauer's moral thought: a *stance* from which we not only reject the pain of others but also rationally criticize our tendency to close ourselves off from the world and separate ourselves from other people by creating a coldness that eventually allows us to constitute conditions under which other people suffer or are actively hurt.

Animality and humanity

Adorno comes the closest to formulating this moral stance in a passage in *Negative Dialectics*: 'the individual is left with no more than the morality for which Kantian ethics – which accords affection, not respect, to animals – can muster only disdain: to try to live so that one may believe himself to have been a good animal.'[69] I believe that we have to connect this claim to a passage in his essay on Kafka to really understand what Adorno suggests here:

> Like his countryman, Gustav Mahler, Kafka sides with the deserters. Instead of human dignity, the supreme bourgeois concept, there emerges in him the salutary recollection of the similarity between man and animal, an idea upon which a whole group of his narratives thrives. Immersion in the inner space of individuation, which culminates in such self-contemplation, stumbles upon the principle of individuation, the postulation of the self by the self, officially sanctioned by philosophy, the mythic defiance. The subject seeks to make amends by abandoning this defiance. Kafka does not glorify the world through subordination; he resists it through nonviolence. Faced with the latter, power must acknowledge itself as that which it is, and it is on this fact alone that he counts.[70]

This complex passage shows us that the notion of 'animality' plays two different roles in the line 'having been a good animal': a parodying and an exemplary role.

The first role is based on a radicalization of tendencies that already exist in the modern world. Instead of clinging to a notion of dignity, following from the idea that every individual, as an individual, is an end in itself, Kafka's stories – *The Metamorphosis* is probably the most famous of these, and in the conclusion to this book I briefly discuss *A Report to an Academy* – revolve around the border between human and animal, often crossing it, thereby confronting the self with the *principium individuationis* on which its individuality rests and which is supposed to differentiate it from the animal. Unlike Schopenhauer, after all, who understands the *principium individuationis* as the result of the irrationally structured world both human and non-human animals perceive – the world-as-representation – Adorno links the constitution of the self to the socially mediated rational self-reflection that enables human beings to elevate themselves out of nature by way of a process that, as we have seen in Chapter 6, evolved into an irrational domination of nature.

Kafka's stories confront us with an extreme version of these ideas: in Adorno's view, they unmask the irrational and violent character of a faculty of reason that declares itself to be 'pure' and of the accompanying notion of an autonomous individual that believes itself to be absolutely independent. They do this by parodying these ideas as follows: the subject turns so violently against itself that it destroys the pillars on which its individuality rests and becomes an animal.[71] Absolute autonomy herewith turns into absolute domination; the freedom that the subject thinks it has achieved in the modern world turns into unfreedom; individuality turns into social determination.

With the line 'having been a good animal' Adorno follows Kafka and explores the border between humans and animals as well, referring to sparks of compassion with suffering creatures that he deliberately provides with an animalistic quality. His moral philosophy hereby reflects the wrongness of the status quo by parodying its character.

But this line also has an exemplary dimension, which is entwined with its parodying dimension. In Adorno's view, animals teach us humility by forcing us to understand ourselves not as fundamentally and categorically different from them. Clinging to the idea that there is a fundamental gap between human and non-human animals overlooks the fact that we are embodied subjects and that our minds are entwined with our corporeal impulses and experiences, as discussed above. It follows from a neurotic and hostile need to completely and categorically distance oneself from nature, a need that transforms itself into a need for the domination of nature. Our kinship with animals, in other words, forces us to look critically at the faculty of reason and prohibits us from celebrating it as a *pure* faculty that, tied to the *principium individuationis*, elevates us *completely* out of nature. This is what animals teach us: a critical and humble understanding of ourselves and the faculty of reason. Jean Améry, whose observations on pain I discussed above, insightfully puts this idea into words as follows by looking at the notion of 'enlightenment':

> The concept of enlightenment must not be too restricted methodologically, for, as I understand it, it embraces more than just logical deduction and empirical verification, but rather, beyond these two, the will and the ability to speculate phenomenologically, to empathize, to approach the limits of reason. Only when we fulfil the law of enlightenment and at the same time transcend it do we reach intellectual realms in which ratio does not lead to shallow rationalism.[72]

Rationality can only be defended, Adorno suggests in line of Améry, if we do not uncritically put it on a pedestal but emphasize its limitations and origins without rejecting it completely.

The observation that the line 'having been a good animal' can both be read as parodying a state in which people are reduced to an animalistic existence *and* as positively referring to the virtue of humility that animals teach us, implies that the moral stance that follows from

Adorno's thought is both critical and exemplary in nature as well. It revolves around a radical critique of social, cultural and psychological mechanisms but at the same time affirms an attitude of humility and openness towards otherness. It rejects the dominating tendencies of reason, but embraces its self-critical abilities.

Conclusion

We have seen that Adorno develops a moral philosophy that arises as a response to a specific, historical situation. Its normative basis consists of an almost ungraspable bodily rejection of the suffering of others, sparking lines like 'Auschwitz should not repeat itself' or 'there should be no atom bomb', rejecting specific phenomena.[73] Nevertheless, his moral philosophy carries further than just these historical events: following our rejection of specific kinds of suffering in specific situations, Adorno develops a moral stance that not only revolves around more general lines like 'Thou shalt not inflict pain' or Benjamin's 'While there is a beggar, there is a myth', but also around the virtue of modesty and the notion of fallibility, ideas that he links to rational critique. Our rejection of suffering, in other words, may spark a self-critical way of thinking, of reflecting on the society in which we live and the tendencies that drive our selves, which results in a radical resistance against the status quo.[74]

This means that Adorno's moral philosophy functions as a critical perspective on a wide range of social phenomena: it forces us to critically reflect on fear of otherness, resulting in racism or discrimination, or on technological and industrialized ways of approaching the lives of others. But it also criticizes the reduction of people to their (suffering) bodies, which robs them of their individuality and particularity. Adorno's moral thought furthermore warns as that we should not hide behind the *principium individuationis* and build up rationalized walls between ourselves and others. His thought introduces a radical egalitarianism that springs from a concern with the vulnerability to pain of every bodily being.

My above-developed interpretation does not imply that Adorno's moral philosophy is not weak or unproblematic: we have seen that it finds its normative basis in rather vague feelings of compassion that people, more often than not, do not experience any more in a social whole that is described as completely overpowering.[75] Furthermore, its normative basis – a bodily spark of compassion that tells us that pain is wrong – is understood by him at the same time as the addendum that forces the subject into action and pushes it out of its passivity: fact and value come very close in his moral philosophy.

Another problematic aspect is that Adorno's reflections on the way in which the wrongness of reality influences (the possibility of) constructing moral principles gravely damages the normative force of his moral philosophy and, eventually, the notion of responsibility. This can be illustrated by his discussion of punishing 'the torturers of Auschwitz'. In *Negative Dialectics* Adorno analyses how the possibility of punishing these torturers is 'falsified' because the principles on which those punishments would be based are always already 'compromised by the same principle on which the killers were acting'.[76] In that sense, the wrongness of the whole in which we live makes it impossible to formulate a moral law or principle on which such a punishment can be based without in some way or another affirming that same wrong whole. On the one hand, this means that these torturers cannot be held responsible, since they were products of a radically distorted and false whole.[77] On the other hand, however, they cannot be let go unpunished. These two opposing ideas represent an objective, social antinomy.

Adorno herewith comes close to Schopenhauer again. We have seen that the latter completely removes freedom from the realm of morality, arguing that we can only feel responsible for our characters since they spark our actions, while at the same time claiming that these characters are unchangeable and that guilt revolves around the wish to be someone else. To a certain extent, Adorno's observations on the distorting and overpowering nature of the modern world undermine the notion of responsibility in a similar fashion: if this world only brings unfreedom and distorts our moral faculties, then how are we responsible for our actions and not mere products of the context in which we live? Again, this shared emphasis on unfreedom, determinism and irresponsibility forms one of the reasons why Lukács made both Schopenhauer and Adorno take up residence in the Grand Hotel Abyss.

Unlike Schopenhauer's ahistorical metaphysics, however, the historical nature of Adorno's moral observations allows him to claim that the fragmented and damaged nature of his moral philosophy is a reflection of the fragmented and damaged nature of modernity: the above-discussed problem of responsibility, in other words, reflects a social, objective problem. In a social and cultural whole in which the subject finds itself in a different relationship with nature, other people and its own body, morality does not have to revolve around a bodily rejection of pain and suffering, or around abhorrence of human constructions like death camps or the atom bomb, Adorno suggests. Furthermore, we could read his analysis of the problem of responsibility as referring to the idea that only as a community can we truly be moral: if society itself is responsible for the evil that people do instead of these individuals themselves, then it is society as a whole that needs to be changed to constitute a morally right world.[78] In Chapter 10 I return to Adorno's ideas on the constitution of a good society.

As long as this does not happen, however, we have to rely on the ungraspable and fragmented moral addendum.[79] And as long as Schopenhauer's metaphysical monism reflects the unfreedom of the modern world, moral philosophy revolves for an important part around *Mitleid*, as Schopenhauer himself claimed in an ahistorical manner. Adorno's references to the phenomenon of compassion hereby reflect a social antinomy: on the one hand, compassion is not sufficient to form the basis of a stable moral philosophy. On the other hand, it is the only moral experience left, in his view.[80] As critical responses to the status quo, Adorno's descriptions of the moral addendum force us to look at the world in a specific way and to ask ourselves the following basic question: why do we keep inflicting pain, actively or passively, on other vulnerable bodily beings that, if inflicted upon ourselves, we would reject with all our force? It is this question that Adorno's moral philosophy forces its readers to confront, as long as unnecessary suffering exists.

9
The Road to Salvation

Introduction

The Portuguese poet Fernando Pessoa wrote under different pseudonyms, which he dubbed 'heteronyms'.[1] Each of these heteronyms has its own biography and represents a different philosophy. One of Pessoa's most famous heteronyms is Alberto Caeiro, who developed a peculiar materialism. His poems express the idea that, ultimately, human beings are bodies, and revolve around the need to escape the world that the subject experiences – a world permeated with desires, strivings, ideas, thoughts and plans – and 'become' the material body.

Caeiro tried to describe nature, including the body, as 'untainted' by the subjective and, in his view, false perspective of experience. He struggled, however, with the problematic aspect of this view, originating in the impossibility of objectively describing the body as an object in a world-of-objects.

Conceptualizing an experience of nature, after all, elevates it out of nature and thereby fails to grasp that which makes this nature into the 'other' of conceptuality. As Richard Zenith puts this in his introduction to a collection of Pessoa's poems: 'Caeiro claimed to be "the only poet of Nature," but his vision of nature was ideal, his appreciation of it abstract, and his poetry is almost pure philosophy. To talk about seeing things directly is tantamount to no longer seeing them.'[2] Caeiro himself was not blind to this problem, poetically criticizing materialism as a paradoxical doctrine as follows: 'You say, sick philosopher, every philosopher, that this is materialism / But how can this be materialism, if materialism is a philosophy'.[3]

Caeiro's poems revolve around the attempt to conceptually overcome the conceptual, to find transcendence *through* oneself: 'All the knowledge there is of things / Was never something I could seize like a thing. / If science aspires to be true, / What truer science than that of things without science?'[4] They express the mystical longing to overcome oneself and to dissolve into an experience in which one, paradoxically, does not experience anymore: a manner of being that is not found in death but that can be understood as a subjectless, 'objective awareness'.

In *Willing and Unwilling* Julian Young observes about Schopenhauer's arguments for pessimism: 'Schopenhauer not only propounds the argument, but also, albeit unemphatically, mitigates its apparent inexorability by hinting at methods of escape.'[5] This chapter revolves around that which Caeiro expresses as the experience of a 'true reality', as a 'science without science', an idea which I will discuss regarding Schopenhauer's 'method of escape': his analysis of salvation. Furthermore, it revolves around the seemingly impossible attempt to put the nature of this utopian experience, bordering on the mystical, into words.

Eternal peace

Incommunicable experiences

In the second half of *The World as Will and Representation* Schopenhauer develops the idea that one can completely extinguish the Will 'within' oneself, which results in an experience of nothingness that forms the ultimate 'method of escape' that his philosophy offers: salvation. This means that his thought is not only driven by the quest to analyse, explain and ground our existence and the ways in which we perceive and experience the world, it is also therapeutic in nature.

Schopenhauer defines this state of salvation as 'an unshakable peace, a deep calm and inward serenity', as an existence in which one is 'freed from all care and anxiety for ever'.[6] In this state the self disappears: it has no ideas, thoughts, strivings, hopes or ideals anymore. It does not experience a world-as-representation, since the boundaries between 'inside' and 'outside', between subject and object have dissolved. It does not suffer either, since all striving has been quietened down and the body has been overcome. The self 'floats', as it were, in a state of nothingness.

Schopenhauer understands this experience of nothingness as the silence that religions and mystical traditions revolve around.[7] Salvation, he writes, is 'denoted by the names of ecstasy, rapture, illumination, union with God, and so on. But such a state cannot really be called knowledge, since it no longer has the form of subject and object; moreover, it is accessible only to one's own experience that cannot be further communicated'.[8] Indeed, he continually stresses that this 'deliverance from a world whose whole existence presented itself to us as suffering'[9] can only be described *negatively*, as a 'transition into empty nothingness'.[10] This forces the philosopher to resort to 'mystical and metaphorical language' because 'it is the only language in which anything can be said about the wholly transcendent theme':[11]

> [T]rue salvation lies in the denial of the will, ... all religions at their highest point end in mysticism and mysteries, that is to say, in darkness and veiled obscurity. These really indicate a blank spot for knowledge, the point where all knowledge necessarily ceases. Hence for thought this can be expressed only by negations.[12]

Salvation has to be lived through, in other words, since philosophy is unable to describe it and since it is categorically different from the world we 'normally' experience and perceive.

Schopenhauer's philosophy herewith results in a critique of the inadequacy of philosophy, which reminds one of the way in which Alberto Caeiro attempts in his poems to conceptually express an experience that, paradoxically, cannot be put into words. His thought ends in 'non-thought' and the ultimate method of escape that his theory provides is non-theoretical. In Schopenhauer's words: 'when my teaching reaches its highest point, it assumes a negative character, and so ends with a negation', adding that 'it is precisely here that the mystic proceeds positively, and therefore, from this point, nothing is left but mysticism'.[13] Within Schopenhauer's thought, philosophy crashes against its own walls, coming up 'against insoluble problems everywhere, as against the wall of our prison',[14] walls over which it can only leap in silence.[15]

Intuitive knowledge

These references to the possibility of salvation, based on a denial of the Will, represent a complete shift within Schopenhauer's philosophy. Whereas he continually emphasizes the idea, as we have seen in Chapters 3, 4 and 7, that everything that exists is a manifestation of Will, that both human and non-human animals are completely unfree, and that we are destined to live a life filled with pain and suffering, he now claims that it is possible to quieten down and eventually annihilate that which we essentially are, leaving behind our striving nature, our corporeality and, eventually, our individuality.

But this introduces a problem: how can I reach salvation if all of my acts are products of my individual Will? How can I, in other words, quieten down my individual Will if this can only be done through acts of willing? The mystical conclusion to Schopenhauer's philosophy appears to be nothing but a crippling paradox.[16]

Schopenhauer's answer to these questions revolves around the notion of 'intuitive knowledge'. Once we have intuitively – not rationally – grasped the nature of ourselves and the world around us, our individual Will starts withering away, Schopenhauer observes. He therefore characterizes salvation as follows: 'Happiness and unhappiness have vanished; we are no longer the individual: that is forgotten; we are only pure subjects of knowledge.'[17] He also refers to this knowledge in a passage in which he characterizes his philosophy as a whole:

> Thus it may be that the inner nature of holiness, of self-renunciation, of mortification of one's own will, of asceticism, is here for the first time expressed in abstract terms and free from everything mythical, as denial of the *will-to-live*, which appears after the complete knowledge of its own inner being has become for it the quieter of all willing.[18]

We have to gain insight into the way of the world and our role in it, in other words, to be able to deny this role and that which drives us.

Schopenhauer describes three ways to acquire this 'pure knowledge', three roads to salvation: aesthetic contemplation, morality and voluntary self-denial. In the following I want to discuss these roads and show how they each embody different stages of salvation, contributing in different ways to that which Schopenhauer seeks to grasp with his complex idea of 'intuitive knowledge'. This discussion will be descriptive in nature; I will look more critically at Schopenhauer's ideas on salvation after this overview of the three roads to salvation.

Schopenhauer's aesthetic theory

In the third book of *The World as Will and Representation* Schopenhauer develops his aesthetic theory. Works of art, he argues, are able to represent or objectify something that philosophy cannot put into words, providing us with brief moments of the above-discussed blissful experience.

The importance that Schopenhauer attributes to the arts is reflected by the fact that he even uses the word 'pleasure' regarding our perception of works of art. Whereas he, as I have shown in Chapter 4, mainly refers with this concept to an *absence* of striving and desiring, it is only in passages on the 'subjectless knowledge' that, in his view, is provided by works of art that *positive* descriptions of pleasure are found.[19] In the first volume of his chief work, for example, he describes the 'delight in the mere knowledge of perception as such',[20] and in its second volume he refers to the 'state of pure objectivity of perception' that makes one 'positively happy'.[21]

In the following I will discuss three aspects of Schopenhauer's analysis of aesthetics: his interpretation of Plato's Ideas, his ideas on tragic art, and his analysis of music. In Chapter 10 we will see that several of these aspects return in Adorno's aesthetic theory.

Platonic Ideas

Schopenhauer's analysis of the arts rests mainly on a peculiar interpretation of Plato. As discussed in Chapter 3, Schopenhauer argues that Plato's dualism between a world of eternal Ideas on the one hand and a world of mere shadows on the other is not unlike the dualism between *noumenon* and *phenomenon* developed by Kant.

We will see that this introduction of Plato's dualism is peculiar. Some have argued that it forms an unnecessary addition to Schopenhauer's philosophy as a whole and should therefore be ignored. Others have defended it as belonging to the core of his philosophy.[22]

Schopenhauer argues that artworks do not express 'particular things, events, change or plurality'[23] but the Ideal essence of the objects that they represent: when viewing a work of art, he claims, the subject perceives the object depicted by that artwork in a 'purely objective manner', referring with 'objectivity' to 'disinterestedness'.[24] He bases these observations on the idea that our perception of the world is almost always guided and influenced by the Will 'inside of us', that is, by emotions, needs, desires and inclinations. We almost always perceive objects, in other words, *in relation to the Will*; as components of possible *motives*: they may trigger needs, desires and drives, possibly resulting in actions. Since artworks do not appeal to the Will as 'regular' and particular objects do, Schopenhauer argues, 'the Ideas of things appeal to us more easily from the work of art than from reality'.[25] It is in this disinterestedness that beauty is found, in Schopenhauer's analysis: 'everything is beautiful so long as it does not concern us.'[26]

This does not mean that beauty is restricted to works of art, only that artworks are beautiful as long as they stand in no relationship to the Will. Furthermore, this definition of beauty does not imply that artworks cannot trigger the Will inside of an individual – a painting of food can, for example, make a hungry person want to eat. However, if this happens, Schopenhauer's argument implies, this person does not view the depicted food in an Ideal sense but in a particular one, and does not find the painting beautiful. As a primary example, Schopenhauer mentions the moon: we find the moon beautiful, he argues, and describe its beauty so often in poems and songs because it stands in no relationship to the Will.[27]

Schopenhauer defines this 'Ideal essence' that artworks embody rather vaguely and in different ways. He links Plato's dualism between Ideas and the world we perceive to his own dualism between the world-as-will and the world-as-representation as follows: 'if for us the will is the *thing-in-itself*, and the *Idea* is the immediate objectivity of that will at a definite grade, then we find Kant's thing-in-itself and Plato's Idea ... to be, not exactly identical, but yet very closely relateds.'[28] Being the 'objectivity of the Will at a definitive grade', Schopenhauer also refers to the Idea as the object's 'character', as '*species rerum*', as its 'unchangeable form' and as the 'purely objective element of phenomena'.[29]

In some way or another, Schopenhauer herewith argues, the disinterestedness with which a subject perceives a work of art allows it to view the *essence* of this object, which 'exists' as an unchangeable Idea 'in-between' the unknowable in-itself of the world-as-will and the objectivity of the world-as-representation. In other words: if we succeed in perceiving an object without in any way experiencing desires, needs and drives that make this particular object interesting to us as particular, willing creatures, it loses its particularity and individuality and we view its unchangeable nature.

It is difficult to understand precisely what position these Ideas hold within Schopenhauer's dualism between world-as-will and world-as-representation. Schopenhauer departs from Plato when he argues that Ideas are not objects of thought but objects of perception. In his view, Ideas are close to the in-itself but 'not yet the essence of the thing-in-itself'.[30] Confusingly, Schopenhauer even claims that Ideas exist in reality since they form the eternal aspect of that which makes a species into a species and an individual member of a species into a manifestation of this species, again stating that Ideas are therefore not the same as concepts.[31]

Schopenhauer couples this 'viewing' of Platonic Ideas not only to a change in the perception of the object but also to a fundamental change in the perceiving subject *itself*. Arguing that our consciousness can be filled with two 'things' – ourselves (that is, ourselves as Will) on the one hand, and objects in the world around us on the other – he claims that the more we focus on the second, the less we are concerned with the first. And this means that in those moments in which we are absorbed by works of art, we turn away from our selves completely.

Combined with his above-discussed observation that when we are absorbed in works of art we elevate ourselves above our existence as creatures defined by Will, Schopenhauer concludes that art allows the subject to become 'no longer an individual, for in such perception the individual has lost himself; he is pure will-less, painless timeless subject of knowledge'.[32] When absorbed in a work of art, in other words, the individual has lost all awareness of him- or herself – and thereby all awareness of him- or herself as a striving and suffering being – and is filled completely with a Will-less contemplation of the artwork.

Schopenhauer defines this contemplation as 'knowledge', since through it we come to *know* the Ideal and objective essence of the depicted object, while at the same time being 'disconnected', as it were, from our particular existence 'in' a world defined by Will. And since Ideas are not the same as concepts and, in some way or another, really 'exist' in his view, Schopenhauer's interpretation of Plato allows him to argue that this knowledge is not rational or conceptual in nature but *intuitive*: it consists of a leaving behind of one's individual mind and an elevation to a higher level on which one becomes 'that one eye of the world which looks out from all knowing creatures'[33] and grasps the nature of the world intuitively.

It is this 'will-less knowing' that constitutes the first road to salvation Schopenhauer discusses. He claims that it can be regarded as 'an act of self-denial'[34] since the individual, willing subject ceases to be in moments of aesthetic contemplation. He adds, however, that 'it must at once be observed that it is not a question of a lasting emancipation, but merely a brief hour of rest, of an exceptional, and in fact only momentary, release from the service of the will'.[35] In Schopenhauer's view, this escape from the Will nevertheless plays an extremely important role in our lives, allowing us to be 'transported' to a different realm:

> For at the moment when, torn from the will, we have given ourselves up to pure, will-less knowing, we have stepped into another world, so to speak, where everything that moves our will, and thus violently agitates us, no longer exists. This liberation of knowledge shifts us as wholly and completely above all this as do sleep and dreams.[36]

The subject that has reached this state of salvation has overcome its violent tendencies, its need to grasp the world and to dominate it. It no longer perceives the world in relation to that which it wants and needs, but in an objective, Ideal state.

Tragic art

This brings us to tragic art, which holds a special position in Schopenhauer's philosophy. Since every art-form represents an Idea, in his view, he argues that tragic plays and tragic poetry objectify 'the Idea of man, an Idea which has the peculiarity of expressing itself in highly individual characters'.[37] Following his pessimistic conclusions regarding the state of the world and the human condition, this 'Idea of man' revolves around the observation that human beings are destined to suffer and that this suffering is often caused by human beings themselves. Schopenhauer therefore specifically praises tragedy that 'shows us the greatest misfortune not as an exception, not as something brought about by rare circumstances or by monstrous characters, but as something that arises easily and spontaneously out of the actions and characters of men, as something almost essential to them.'[38]

Tragic art herewith allows us to objectively view the Idea of human beings as manifestations of Will, as mere cogs in metaphysical machine of blind striving: 'the unspeakable pain, the wretchedness and misery of mankind, the triumph of wickedness, the scornful mastery of chance, and the irretrievable fall of the just and the innocent are all here presented to us: and here is to be found a significant hint as to the nature of the world and of existence'.[39]

But tragic art does more, according to Schopenhauer. Tragic heroes – and in this context he mentions Gretchen in *Faust*, Hamlet's friend Horatio, Palmira in Voltaire's *Mohammed, The Maid of Orleans* and Schiller's *The Bride of Messina*[40] – show us how, after a life filled with suffering and with senseless striving that knows no satisfaction, a process of self-denial can be set in motion. Tragic heroes, he argues, are 'purified by suffering' and reach a state in which they are able to turn away from that which has driven them all their lives: the will-to-live.

Not only does tragic art provide us with an example of ways to turn away from the Will, it also enables us to perceive the suffering that takes place in the world without suffering ourselves, which means that tragedy addresses its readers or spectators in a unique manner, confronting them with what they essentially are. To a certain extent, Schopenhauer herewith suggests that the knowledge that arises from perceiving a tragic play rests on an identification of the spectator with the tragic hero, a process that does not take place when perceiving, for example, a still life depicting an apple. This difference may function as an explanation of the observation that tragedy often grasps its spectators in an intense manner, making them shudder as bodily beings at the sight of the horrors that are depicted, responding to the fate of the tragic hero in an almost compassionate manner.

It has therefore been suggested that Schopenhauer is implying that the knowledge people gain by reading tragic poetry or by watching a tragic play is *cognitive* and *rational* in nature rather than intuitive; it follows from a realization people arrive at as reflective individuals.[41] Tragic art, this interpretation goes, results in knowledge about the world because it addresses its readers or spectators not as pure, will-less subjects but *as* manifested Will, *as* bodies, while at the same time as creatures capable of cognitive insight.

Even though these suggestions emphasize an important aspect of tragic art, I believe it should be kept in mind that Schopenhauer clearly refers to this kind of art as representing the 'Idea' of humanity. Nevertheless, his emphasis on the example set by tragic heroes does imply that we, as spectators, are involved in tragic plays: we feel compassion with its heroes and experience relief when they eventually manage to deny their will. In this sense, the spectators or readers of tragic art are both involved and uninvolved: they intuitively grasp the 'Idea of man', which requires distance and passivity, but reach this state by actively empathizing with the fate of tragic heroes and by rationally connecting it to their own existence as striving and suffering beings.

Music

The special place that tragic art occupies within Schopenhauer's aesthetics brings us to music, which he characterizes as the highest of the arts; as a 'universal language' that is 'instantly understood by everyone'.[42] In his view, music forms the most 'universal language' because it is not conceptual in nature and can therefore show us the 'innermost kernel of things' in a way that the concept cannot, because it only grasps the 'stripped-off outer shell of things'[43] and is different in each language. Furthermore, he claims that music forms the most 'real' or 'direct' *representation* of the Will.

Like the other arts, he argues, music is a representation, but its non-conceptual and unique nature manages to come extremely close to Will *itself*. The melodic movements of music and the different tones and layers within musical compositions reflect the movements of the Will, striving for life on the countless levels and realms of nature – from the waves of the sea to moving glaciers, from bacteria to plants, from animals to human beings: 'the nature of melody is a constant digression and deviation from the keynote in a thousand ways.... In all these ways, melody expresses the many different forms of the will's efforts.'[44]

Listening to a symphony, Schopenhauer implies, is like walking through a rainforest, noticing how on every level life is striving; how the most beautiful and strange organisms have developed at the most unlikely places; living, breathing, striving without reflection or inner purpose: blind Will, fighting for life, crystallized into forms and shapes that exceed the imagination.

Indeed, Schopenhauer emphasizes the close connection between the metaphysics of music and the metaphysics of nature, stating that 'we can regard the phenomenal world, or nature, and music as two different expressions of the same thing'[45] and even adds that 'we could just as well call the world embodied music as embodied will.'[46] Enjoying the beauty of nature, Schopenhauer suggests, is similar to enjoying the beauty of music: both consist of the experience of wonder at a world defined by endless movements and strivings, by a blind but all-overpowering force.

This brings us to Schopenhauer's definition of the 'sublime'. Unlike beauty, which he links to a calm and will-less perception of the 'true nature of the world', he argues that the sublime is constituted *violently* when one is torn away from one's individual nature and one's needing and striving character. Like the contemplation of beauty, however, this experience results in a state of pure knowledge, in his view:

> [W]ith the sublime, that state of pure knowing is obtained first of all by a conscious and violent tearing away from the relations of the same object to the will which are recognized as unfavourable, by a free exaltation, accompanied by consciousness, beyond the will and the knowledge related to it.[47]

I return below to the complex nature of this 'consciousness beyond Will'. For now, it is important to emphasize that, in Schopenhauer's view, music allows us to overview the nature and essence of the world at a *distant* but, paradoxically, also *involved* way:

> Only in this way does music never cause us actual suffering, but still remains pleasant even in its most painful chords; and we like to hear in its language the secret history of our will and of all its stirrings and strivings with their many different delays, postponements, hindrances, and afflictions, even in the most sorrowful melodies. On the other hand, where in real life and its terrors our *will itself* is that which is roused and tormented, we are then not concerned with tones and their numerical relations; on the contrary, we ourselves are now the vibrating string that is stretched and plucked.[48]

This reference to the 'secret history of our will' implies that music, like tragic art, not only revolves around an intuitive grasping of the nature of the world, but also around a *recognition* of that which we essentially are: when listening to music, we feel that what is represented is also what drives us as living, embodied beings. Music, Schopenhauer therefore writes, represents 'human wiling in general, in so far as it is expressed universally through its objectivity, the human body'.[49]

To a certain extent, this even means that Schopenhauer claims that music allows us grasp our 'oneness' with the essence of the universe: it allows us to know intuitively that, essentially, we are not individuals but mere parts of an overpowering and blind whole with which we realize our unity once we have thrown off our individual willing.[50] Music, after all, represents not individual willing, like fear or desire, Schopenhauer writes, but 'human willing in general'. In his discussion of the arts, Schopenhauer indeed translates the Sanskrit *Mahāvākya* 'Tat tvam asi' not as 'this art thou' – as he normally does – but as 'this living thing art thou'.[51]

Even though Schopenhauer emphasizes the idea that music forms a representation of the Will, these ideas about experiencing a certain kinship with the essence of the universe do provide his theory of music with a special aura: again, unlike viewing a painting of an apple, for example, music allows us to come really close to the nature of the universe and thereby to experience a certain 'distant involvement' with this nature. It addresses us *as that which we are* and does not only allow us to contemplate the Ideal essence of objects: it confronts us, as individuals, with the pre-individualistic source of our existence and our suffering.

Compassion and self-denial

Compassion

Whereas aesthetic contemplation, in all its different forms, provides 'only momentary' a 'release from the service of the will',[52] Schopenhauer describes two other roads to salvation that may result in a more long-lasting state of salvation. He discusses the first of these two roads in the last paragraphs of the first volume of *The World as Will and Representation*. There, he argues that a profound concern for and meditation on the suffering of one's fellow creatures not only transforms one into a self-less and moral person – as discussed in Chapter 7 – but may, in certain cases, also result in a person in whom the Will is 'quietened down' and eventually 'dies', resulting in what he portrays as the most desirable state of existence we are able to attain as human animals. Schopenhauer expresses this idea as follows:

> If that veil of Maya, the *principium individuationis*, is lifted from the eyes of a man to such an extent that he no longer makes the egoistical distinction between himself and the person of others, but takes as much interest in the sufferings of other individuals as in his own, and thus is not only benevolent and charitable in the highest degree, but even ready to sacrifice his own individuality whenever several others can be saved thereby, then it follows automatically that such a man, recognizing in all beings his own true and innermost self, must also regard the endless sufferings of all that lives as his own, and thus takes upon himself the pain of the whole world. [...T]hat knowledge of the whole, of the inner nature of the thing-in-itself..., becomes the *quieter* of all and every willing.[53]

A change may take place, in other words, 'in' people who are affected to an enormous extent by the suffering of other people. Again, Schopenhauer defines this change mainly as the acquisition of *knowledge*, of an *awareness* of the nature of the universe that is accompanied by a withering away of the self. This knowledge is not rational, logical or propositional in nature: it is not gained through reasoning or *caused* by anything. It arises in an *intuitive* and rather *passive* manner in the person who takes the suffering of other beings to his or her heart like they are his or her own, piercing through the *principium individuationis* and elevating him- or herself to a mystical state in which he or she is aware of the 'great truth' that 'all is one'.[54] Schopenhauer describes this process as follows:

> Every purely beneficent act, every instance of wholly and truly disinterested help, which as such has another's distress as its motive, is, if we probe the matter to the bottom, really a mysterious action. It is practical mysticism insofar as it ultimately springs from the same knowledge that constitutes the essence of all mysticism proper. In no other way can it be truly explained.[55]

It is from the perspective of this intuitive knowledge that, in Schopenhauer's view, 'virtue' arises: 'the intuitive knowledge that recognizes in another's individuality the same inner nature as in one's own'.[56] The practical mystic 'sees himself in all places simultaneously, and withdraws. His will turns about; it no longer affirms its own inner nature, mirrored in the phenomenon, but denies it. The phenomenon by which this becomes manifest is the transition from virtue to *ascetism*'.[57]

Even though the state of being that Schopenhauer describes borders on the realm of morality, its mystical nature makes it into more than that. In Chapters 4 and 7 we have seen that, in Schopenhauer's view, morality is based on 'moments' of compassion that are constantly threatened and dominated by egotistic tendencies. We have furthermore seen that he is ambivalent about the extent to which someone who experiences compassion truly leaves his own skin behind. He claims, for example: 'at every moment we remain clearly conscious that he is the sufferer, not we; and it is precisely in his person, not in ours, that we feel the suffering, to our grief and sorrow. We suffer with him and hence in him; we feel his pain as his, and do not imagine that it is ours.'[58] Schopenhauer therefore describes moral virtues as 'only a step towards' 'the ultimate end'.[59] Once we enter the metaphysical and mystical sphere, he suggests, this latter duality truly dissolves, elevating us to a level in which we see through the *principium individuationis* and grasp the essence of our existence:

> [F]rom this point of view, it might occur to us that the really proper address between one man and another should be, instead of Sir, Monsieur, and so on, 'Leidensgefährte'...'compagnon de misères', 'my fellow-sufferer'. However strange this may sound, it...reminds us of that most necessary thing, tolerance, patience, forbearance, and love of one's neighbour, which everyone needs and each of us, therefore, owes to another.[60]

It is important to notice that, like his descriptions of aesthetic contemplation, the tone of Schopenhauer's mystical observations is radically different from the way he describes other aspects of life. Not only does 'practical mysticism' revolve around love and tolerance, he even refers to an 'enlargement of the heart' in this context: 'the knowledge that every living thing is just as much our own inner being-in-itself as is our own person, extends our interest to all that lives; and in this way the heart is enlarged.'[61]

Ascetism

This brings us to the third road to salvation that Schopenhauer describes: *active* self-denial, which is not moral in nature and therefore not focused on other beings. Instead, it is directed at *oneself* as a striving creature. In this context, Schopenhauer mentions 'voluntary and complete chastity',[62] a denial of sexual satisfaction, poverty, a 'constant mortification of the will',[63] and even self-castigation and self-torture. These practices are understood as 'killing' the Will within oneself by extinguishing, impeding or denying one's bodily impulses and feelings in what Schopenhauer calls a 'constant struggle with temptations'.[64] To illustrate this radical idea, he refers at several places to saints and mystics found 'among the Christians, and even more among the Hindus and Buddhists, and even among the believers of other religions'.[65]

The hitherto discussed roads eventually lead, according to Schopenhauer, to a definitive state of salvation:

> [T]he denial of the will-to-live...always proceeds from that quieter of the will; and this is the knowledge of its inner conflict and its essential vanity, expressing themselves in the suffering of all that lives. The difference, that we have described as two paths, is whether that knowledge is called forth by suffering which is merely and simply *known* and freely appropriated by our seeing through the *principium individuationis*, or by suffering immediately felt by ourselves.[66]

Whereas egotism, sexual love, self-preservation, eating and drinking are understood as following from an *affirmation* of Will, the three hitherto discussed roads to salvation are each based on a *denial* of Will: they revolve around a perception of the Ideal nature of the world in which the subject abolishes its tendencies to dominate and need and becomes pure, will-less knowledge; around deep compassion with our fellow-sufferers in which the *principium individuationis* is pierced through and the subject overcomes its individualistic nature; or around an active and voluntary destruction of our tendencies and needs, again resulting in a subject that has left its individual Will behind.

Each of these three roads revolves around a negative understanding of the body. In the case of active self-denial, for example, the body is explicitly understood as the seat of the Will and as that which needs to be treated negatively or even aggressively: 'just as he [the self-denier] mortifies the will itself, so does he mortify its visibility, its objectivity, the body.'[67]

The same holds true for his aesthetics. Even though Schopenhauer cannot deny that the senses have to play a role in aesthetic experiences – after all, we have to *see* a painting or *hear* a symphony – he explicitly argues that the body as Will is not excited or triggered when we contemplate art.[68]

In the second volume of the *World as Will and Representation* Schopenhauer states: 'There is only one inborn error, and that is the notion that we exist in order to be happy. It is inborn in us, because it coincides with our existence itself, and our whole being is only its paraphrase, indeed our body is its monogram.'[69] Only by denying or, at least, ignoring this 'monogram' – the body and its inclinations – can we leave this 'inborn error' behind and find peace and calmness, he therefore concludes.

The antagonism of the will with itself

Hurrying back to unconsciousness

But Schopenhauer's discussion of the three roads that lead to salvation has not answered the question how the intuitive knowledge brought about by these roads results in a quietening down of the Will. The key to Schopenhauer's understanding of this process lies in what he calls 'the antagonism of the will with itself',[70] which he describes as follows in his analysis of the tragic heroes that are depicted by tragic art:

> It [this antagonism] becomes visible in the suffering of mankind which is produced partly by chance and error; and these stand forth as the rulers of the world, personified as fate through their insidiousness which appears almost like purpose and intention. In part it proceeds from mankind itself through the self-mortifying efforts of will on the part of individuals, through the wickedness and perversity of most. It is one and the same will, living and appearing in them all, whose phenomena fight with one another and tear one another to pieces. In one individual it appears powerfully, in another more feebly. Here and there it reaches thoughtfulness and is softened more or less by the light of knowledge, until at last in the individual case this knowledge is purified and enhanced by suffering itself. It then reaches the point where the phenomenon, the veil of Maya, no longer deceives it.[71]

Instead of claiming that it is the individual that gains knowledge of the true nature of Will, Schopenhauer argues that it is the Will itself that, *through* the individual, arrives at insight into the antagonisms that constitutes its phenomenal appearance. Schopenhauer suggests that this antagonism is rooted in the observation that the Will, which is endless, timeless and blind *in itself*, is manifested 'in' the world-as-representation in separate forms that not only suffer from their existence as individual beings – they are constantly overcome by strivings and desires that are too 'big' for them because they follow from the Will itself – but that also actively hurt each other in an on-going struggle for survival.

It is the *principium individuationis*, this passage suggests, that constitutes an antagonism of the Will with itself, breaking it up in separate pieces that are destined to suffer and hurt one another in a world structured by time, space and causality. 'At bottom', Schopenhauer claims, as we have seen in Chapter 4, 'we are something that ought not to be'.[72] A similar idea returns in the following passage:

> Awakened to life out of the night of unconsciousness, the will finds itself as an individual in an endless and boundless world, among innumerable individuals, all striving, suffering, and erring; and, as if through a troubled dream, it hurries back to the old unconsciousness. Yet till then its desires are unlimited, its claims inexhaustible, and every satisfied desire gives birth to a new one.[73]

'Normally', Schopenhauer here suggests, the Will does not arrive at this conclusion: manifested as an individual, it is only concerned with its individual strivings and desires, attempting to survive as an individual vessel in which it is destined to be constantly frustrated. However, once it is confronted with the suffering that takes place in the world (through suffering itself or through the 'Idea of man' objectified in tragic art); once it is provided with an understanding of its original unity by way of the phenomenon of compassion or a musical symphony; or once the subject is separated from its individual drives when it is lost in aesthetic contemplation, the Will finally gains knowledge of the antagonism that it contains 'as phenomenon' and of the fact that the individual 'should not be'. The notion of freedom plays an important role in this knowledge, which comes about when the Will realizes that, as thing-in-itself, it is truly free, whereas, as a phenomenon, it is unfree and destined to suffer. This knowledge of the Will's unfreedom 'in' the world-as-representation results in the phenomenon coming 'into a certain contradiction with itself',[74] Schopenhauer writes, through which 'an elimination and self-denial of the will in its most perfect phenomenon is possible, by the will's relating such knowledge to itself'.[75] Then, the individual motives and tendencies that dominate the individual 'in' whom this Will becomes self-aware lose their power, their grip, which results in a quietening down of the will-to-live.[76] Even though this process, in other words, takes place in an individual, this individual itself remains completely passive, Schopenhauer suggests. Still, however, he argues that the observation that this process can take place 'in' human beings means that 'man can certainly be called free, and can thus be distinguished from all other beings'.[77] Only by way of the *human* animal, in other words, can the phenomenon be brought into contradiction with itself: only in human beings can the freedom of an in-itself that lies outside of time, space and causality be contrasted with the unfreedom of a world-as-representation that is structured by these laws. And even though this contradiction is brought about in an individual that remains passive, this *does* mean that such an individual can be characterized as 'free', Schopenhauer claims. As we have already seen in Chapter 4, he herewith again intrinsically links freedom to passivity, and implies that the ability to act has nothing to do with the ability to be free.

The paradox of self-denial

But this idea contains several paradoxes. His emphasis on passivity, for example, is directly contradicted by Schopenhauer's own analyses of asceticism and voluntary self-denial, which suggest that it is possible to *actively* deny one's will. In these cases it is the individual that *wills* not to will; it is not the Will itself withering away from the subject, but the willing subject actively *striving* towards a specific goal. Voluntary self-denial, in other words, can only be thought of as an act of the same Will it seeks to deny.

It could be argued that in individuals who practice asceticism, the self-loathing of the Will has reached such an extreme level that it overpowers the drive to self-preservation and the tendency to flee pain, and therefore even manages to influence the actions of an individual. But this interpretation goes against all of Schopenhauer's own ideas regarding the power of the individual Will and the passive nature of intuitive knowledge.

A second problem is that it remains unclear what precisely happens when the Will turns away from itself 'in' an individual: if one's individual will is quietened down and eventually overcome, what remains of the subject? Does it become one with the Will itself *beyond* the *principium individuationis*? But how is it then able to experience nothingness, peace and freedom if this same Will is the source of our torments? In the last chapter of the first volume of *The World as Will and Representation*, Schopenhauer writes the following about those who have managed to deny the will:

> That we abhor nothingness so much is simply another way of saying that we will life so much, and that we are nothing but this will and know nothing but it alone. But we now turn our glance from our

> own needy and perplexed nature to those who have overcome the world, in whom the will, having reached complete self-knowledge, has found itself again in everything, and then freely denied itself, and who then merely wait to see the last trace of the will vanish with the body that is animated by that trace. Then, instead of the restless pressure and effort; instead of the constant transition from desire to apprehension and from joy to sorrow; instead of never-satisfied and never-dying hope that constitutes the life-dream of the man who wills, we see that peace that is higher than all reason, that ocean-like calmness of the spirit, that deep tranquillity, that unshakeable confidence and serenity, whose mere reflection in the countenance, as depicted by Raphael and Correggio, is a complete and certain gospel. Only knowledge remains; the will has vanished.[78]

On the one hand, Schopenhauer suggests that the Will turns away from its manifestation as an individual and denies only its existence as a particular being. On the other he argues that the Will denies itself *as a whole* once it has 'found itself again in everything'.

According to the first reading, the individual subject dissolves into the Will like a drop of water into the ocean, and experiences an 'ocean-like calmness' that follows from its embeddedness in a larger and free whole, not structured by time, space or causality. According to the second reading, this drop of water evaporates once it has intuitively grasped that, as a drop of water, it is essentially ocean; an endless and blind striving. Once evaporated, it reaches a state of nothingness 'above' this ocean and finds true peace.

The first reading does justice to Schopenhauer's claim that the Will turns away from itself as an individual and that suffering arises only when the Will is 'squeezed' into an individual body and thereby made unfree.[79] Furthermore, this reading answers the question of what the self becomes part of once it has left its individuality behind: everything, after all, is Will, Schopenhauer repeatedly claims.

The second reading does justice to the idea that salvation rests on a complete denial of Will; on the Will reaching knowledge of itself 'through' or 'in' the individual. Furthermore, it affirms Schopenhauer's original ideas about the world-as-representation and the world-as-will, according to which the former is merely the manner in which the subject *perceives* a world that is essentially Will. According to this interpretation, suffering is not caused by the fact that the Will is 'squeezed' into the individual and finds peace and freedom once it leaves this vessel – this would, after all, suggest a different relation between world-as-will and world-as-representation, providing the latter with an ontological status since its structure has the power to influence and shape the former – but because the Will itself is blind and we, as individuals, foolishly expect the world to be defined by purpose, goal and sense. This interpretation, in other words, holds true to Schopenhauer's claim that the essence of the universe is not benevolent, but aimless and cruel.

Given Schopenhauer's emphasis on knowledge and on the experience of nothingness, I want to argue that the second interpretation is the most convincing. This interpretation suggests that once we have reached knowledge of the mythical nature of the *principium individuations* and of the unity of everything that exists, the subject does not long to become part of this unity but completely turns away from it. Salvation, this reading implies, is found in a will-less and bodiless state of consciousness, in a turning away from the ocean of Will by evaporating into nothingness. Schopenhauer's analyses of music and the sublime point in a similar direction: they contain the idea that there is something rewarding, even pleasurable, about the experience of being torn away from one's individual Will and to spectate and know the Will as it is *without* becoming part of it. In the passage quoted above, Schopenhauer describes this experience as 'a free exaltation, accompanied by consciousness, beyond the will and the knowledge related to it'.[80]

Christopher Janaway develops a similar interpretation, which is helpful in this context.[81] He argues that the notion of a 'better consciousness' dominates Schopenhauer's ideas about salvation, which is a consciousness that is completely 'distanced' from the individual and its individual Will, based on a 'seeing through' the *principium individuationis* and on the realization that 'everything is one'.[82] Janaway hereby leans more towards the Platonic than towards the Kantian tendencies of Schopenhauer's thought and, in my view, rightly seeks to do justice to the profound role that art plays in Schopenhauer's philosophy.

This interpretation can be put into words differently: salvation is based on a *phenomenological* shift in the subject. Whereas this subject 'normally' perceives the world as structured by the *principium individuationis*, the knowledge that this principle is an illusion allows the subject to view the world as it is: consisting of endless, blind striving. The Will – not just the individual Will, but the Will in general – then starts withering away and loses its grip on the subject. This process enables this subject to overcome its relations with the world, defined by needs and drives, and to become pure contemplation. It has, in other words, completely changed its way of relating to the world, which allows it to perceive the world without the bonds of Will and to elevate itself to a higher plane of consciousness.

With this emphasis on the phenomenological nature of Schopenhauer's references to Will, we return to my interpretation of his metaphysics and the role it plays in his theory of compassion, developed in Chapter 3. According to this reading, Schopenhauer's notion of Will does not refer to the absolute and unknowable in-itself of the universe, disappearing into overly vague speculations, but it encapsulates experiences of 'otherness' that are related to the experiencing, embodied self. Schopenhauer is first of all concerned, my interpretation goes, with the different ways in which this subject is able to *relate* to the world in which it lives: his most convincing observations regard the bonds between subject and object. And whether these concern the relationship between self and others – either defined by egotism or by compassion – or the relationship between self and world – either defined by strivings or by a subject that has overcome its desires – Schopenhauer's conclusions do not concern ontological changes 'in' the subject, I want to suggest.

Three interpretations

A single thought

Even though I believe that this interpretation provides us with the most convincing overall solution to the problems inherent to Schopenhauer's theory of salvation, it does not solve all of these problems. For example, it leaves the process of *active* and voluntary self-denial unexplained, and is based on the idea that the Will is not all-present or all-powerful. It implicitly accepts the claim that the subject can experience an emptiness beyond the Will: air above the ocean into which the drop of water evaporates. It does not enable us to make sense of Schopenhauer's peculiar theory of Platonic Ideas either: my emphasis on the phenomenological nature of Schopenhauer's observations is not compatible with his ontological claim that these Ideas actually *exist* in some way or another. My interpretation furthermore raises the question: how is the experience of bliss possible if Schopenhauer claims that the boundaries between subject and object have been overcome completely? How can one have experiences in such a state at all?

Another problematic observation is that Schopenhauer seems to deny the naturalistic undertones of most of his observations on the embodied subject: since he often equates the mind to the brain and links his ideas on the primacy of Will to the conclusion that our biology determines our existence, his ideas on overcoming the Will imply that the subject can completely 'disconnect' itself from its body. But how is this possible if this subject is understood as rooted in the brain?

This means that the contradictions on which Schopenhauer's ideas on self-denial are based force us to reject certain parts of his philosophy and preserve others: it is impossible to arrive at a conclusion that is consistent with all of his observations and arguments. Again, Lukács' claim that Schopenhauer's philosophy slides down into 'sophistry'[83] therefore comes to mind, according to which the latter celebrates an uncritical form of mysticism that provides an ontological status to vague feelings of oneness, which collapses once we analyse it rationally and systematically.

This observation, however, contrasts with Schopenhauer's own understanding of his philosophy: in the introduction to *The World as Will and Interpretation* he claims that this work forms the expression of 'one single thought':

> What is to be imparted by [*The World as Will and Representation*] is a single thought. Yet in spite of all my efforts, I have not been able to find a shorter way of imparting that thought than the whole of this book.... *[A] single thought,* however comprehensive, must preserve the most perfect unity. If, all the same, it can be split up into parts for the purpose of being communicated, then the connexion of these parts must once more be organic, i.e., of such a kind that every part supports the whole just as much as it is supported by the whole; a connexion in which no part is first and no part last, in which the whole gains in clearness from every part, and even the smallest part cannot be fully understood until the whole has been first understood.[84]

Schopenhauer's philosophy, he himself claims, should be taken seriously as a systematic whole in which every part matters equally and in which the first sentence leads by a straight argumentative line to the last one.[85]

Since this is obviously not the case, some people have argued that Schopenhauer's theory of salvation should be rejected because it contains too many contradictions and damages the other aspects of his thought.[86] Others have developed more creative interpretations of Schopenhauer's philosophy as a whole.

In the following, I want to look at three of these interpretations, each emphasizing certain interesting aspects of his thought. This will not only allow me to develop an overview of the influence and scope of

Schopenhauer's works, but also to conclude my discussion of his philosophy in this book.

Schopenhauer as an artist

A first interpretation of Schopenhauer's philosophy explicitly departs from his idea that it is the unfolding of 'one single thought'. Instead of presenting a consistent philosophical theory, this interpretation approaches Schopenhauer as developing a meditation on the tensions and paradoxes inherent to our lives as human beings. It implies that, even though Schopenhauer's philosophy is not convincing *as a system*, it is inspiring as a *worldview* or *perspective* that proposes a way of dealing with one's existence as a suffering creature overcome by passions, desires and all-transcending striving, not unlike Alberto Caeiro's attempts to return to descriptions of nature 'as it is' and to leave all goals, plans, feelings, ideas, concepts and reflections behind.

According to this view, his philosophy should be understood as reflecting feelings of powerlessness, of being overcome with passions and desires and with the realization that one is a mere animal in a meaningless world. The paradoxes that his philosophy contains should, in turn, be interpreted as reflecting the inability of the human animal to grasp its own existence, and his aesthetic theory should be read as providing a powerful analysis of the redeeming qualities of the arts. Even though his philosophy is not a systematic whole, this interpretation suggests that it embodies a radical resistance against the world and our place as human beings in it, expressing our struggles, doubts and needs.

It is not surprising that this approach to Schopenhauer's philosophy has mainly been developed by artists or by thinkers that feel closely related to the realm of aesthetics. Maupassant, for example, characterized Schopenhauer as 'the greatest devastator of dreams who ever walked the earth',[87] an idea described as well by Georg Simmel in his classic book on Schopenhauer and Nietzsche:

> The essence and originality of Schopenhauer is related to two important shifts of accent within the philosophical interpretation of the world. First, the will and not 'reason'... is viewed as the radical root of the soul and world. Second, in the wake of all the typically optimistic transfigurations of reality, the deep and irrevocable suffering of the world has finally found its first real and basic expression.[88]

Max Horkheimer develops a similar reading, admiring Schopenhauer for the radical moral ethos his philosophy expresses, an ethos that, in his view, consists of a fundamental resistance against any thinking that deems the world to be 'good' or 'benevolent'. As mentioned in the Introduction to this book, Horkheimer deeply identified with Schopenhauer's concern with suffering and with his attacks on the identitarian philosophical systems developed by the post-Kantian Idealists. In Horkheimer's own words: 'the highest, the most real, the metaphysical being to which philosophers had directed their view, away from the changing world of existing objects, is not at the same time the good. Degrees of reality are not degrees of perfection.'[89]

In light of this interpretation of Schopenhauer, several commentators emphasize the therapeutic aura of the last book of *The World as Will and Representation* and the important influence it has had on authors, painters and playwrights.[90] Examples are Leo Tolstoy and the Dutch author Gerard Reve. Tolstoy cites Schopenhauer extensively in *A Confession*, his autobiographical story concerning his existential crisis,[91] and Reve was deeply influenced by Schopenhauer's ideas on suffering, sexuality, aesthetics and his claim that the ultimate goal of existence is salvation.[92]

Another example is Samuel Beckett. Not only did Beckett recognize his own melancholia in Schopenhauer's philosophy, he also found him to have a therapeutic influence on his suffering and sickness. Gottfriet Büttner writes in an insightful paper on Schopenhauer's influence on Beckett: 'In July 1930 [Beckett] wrote to his friend Thomas MacGreevy: "I am reading Schopenhauer. Everyone laughs at that", and goes on to explain that he is not concerned about whether Schopenhauer "is right or wrong" or whether he is a "good or worthless metaphysician"; instead, he is looking for "an intellectual justification of unhappiness – the greatest that has ever been attempted".'[93] Beckett here explicitly claims that the inconsistency of Schopenhauer's philosophy as a theory is not important once we read him as providing a reflection on our lives as suffering creatures and seek relief from our suffering by empathizing with a mind in whom we recognizes our inner torments. As Beckett states in a letter written from his sickbed:

> I found the only thing I could read was Schopenhauer. Everything else I tried only confirmed the feeling of sickness.... I always knew he was one of the ones that mattered most to me, and it is a pleasure more real than any pleasure for a long time to begin to understand now why it is so. And it is a pleasure also to find a philosopher that can be read like a poet.[94]

The same admiration for Schopenhauer was experienced by the twenty-one-year-old Nietzsche when he purchased Schopenhauer's masterwork in Leipzig 'on impulse' in 1865, finding in it, 'above all, consolation in the face of death'.[95]

Although this is an interesting interpretation of Schopenhauer's works that certainly does justice to an important *aspect* of his thought – an aspect that makes him a rather unique thinker in the history of philosophy – it rests, of course, on the idea that we should not really take Schopenhauer seriously as a philosophical thinker and overlook the observation that Schopenhauer develops arguments and places himself firmly in the philosophical tradition. Nevertheless, this interpretation has been adopted by many, resulting in the fact that Schopenhauer does not play an important role in most academic studies and debates of today.

Stages on life's way

This brings us to a second interpretation of Schopenhauer's thought, which revolves around the idea that *The World as Will and Representation* describes different stages on life's way that each embody a different perspective on life and that follow each other up, guided by a therapeutic logic. Since these stages are each accompanied by a 'deeper' insight into the world, the fact that they contradict each other is not necessarily problematic, this interpretation suggests. The phrase 'stages on life's way', of course, refers to Kierkegaard, who, in several works, describes three ways of relating to the world and other people, which revolve around the realms of aesthetics, ethics and religion.[96]

This interpretation is confirmed by the observation that Schopenhauer pushes every claim – whether it regards the world-as-representation *or* the world-as-will, *or* the idea that we are completely unfree *or* the claim that we *can* reach salvation and freedom – to the ultimate limit, defending each perspective through exaggerations and hyperboles, even going so far as to contradict claims made in earlier or later books. On this approach, we could read the *World as Will and Representation* as follows: as we progress in Schopenhauer's chief work, we ascend, as it were, on a spiral staircase and are led from defences of the objectivity or true nature of the world-as-representation; to the overwhelming and deeper-lying nature of the world-as-will; to several 'methods of escape' that allow us to connect to other living beings; and to ways to overcome the seemingly inescapable nature of our situation as individual creatures.

Julian Young insightfully phrases this development as consisting of the following four 'noble truths': 'the world is my representation; its essence is will, that is to say, suffering; temporary release from suffering is possible through art; permanent release is possible through "denial of the will".'[97] Schopenhauer indeed refers to the Christian idea of 'the natural man' who has to completely *change* his self and thereby elevate himself to another level in order to understand the world in a new way and to eventually experience salvation.[98]

Furthermore, the observation that Schopenhauer resorts to religious metaphors to express the idea that language is meaningless regarding the experience of salvation, does remind one of the importance that the concept of silence plays in *Fear and Trembling*, in which Kierkegaard's pseudonym Johannes de Silentio argues that the relationship between 'the knight of faith' and God is too personal to be expressed in words, constantly suffering from 'the pain of being unable to make himself understandable to others.'[99]

These similarities between Schopenhauer and Kierkegaard, however, are rather superficial and can only be pushed towards a certain point: whereas Kierkegaard understands the silence of the knight of faith, for example, as filled with anxiety, Schopenhauer describes an experience of eternal nothingness, of peace and calm, a state that is desirable and that is the result of an *overcoming* of fear and trembling.

More generally, there are two important problems with this solution to the paradoxes in Schopenhauer's philosophy. First, this interpretation does not do justice to Schopenhauer's claim that he tries to build a system, that he expresses 'one single thought' and that each part of his philosophy is equally important. Schopenhauer indeed argues that his theory of salvation forms the *conclusion* to the observations described in the previous books.[100]

The second problem with this solution is that it does not solve the contradiction *inherent* to what would be its last stage: even if we read the last book of *The World as Will and Representation* as a perspective on its own, we would still end up with the contradiction between Schopenhauer's claim that the self – a manifestation of individual Will – can actively deny the individual Will, and with the problematic nature of the 'space' that the will-less subject occupies.[101]

Schopenhauer as a religious thinker

This Kierkegaardian reading of Schopenhauer's thought brings us to an interpretation that follows religious lines, developed by Gerard Mannion in *Schopenhauer, Religion and Morality: the Humble Path to Ethics*. Mannion seeks to understand Schopenhauer's philosophy as 'fully coherent'[102] while at the same time preserving the idea that one can discern several 'stages' in his philosophy, as discussed above.[103] He does not deny that there are paradoxes inherent to Schopenhauer's thought, but claims that they reflect the paradoxes inherent in most religious forms of thinking:

> Mystery and paradox in Schopenhauer must be understood not as being a mark of despair but ... along the ways in which theologians have tried to define the nature and limits of how we can talk about our understanding (or lack of it) concerning God, ultimate reality or the thing-in-itself.[104]

Following the above-discussed problem that it remains unclear 'where' the self ends up once it has denied the Will and experiences pure nothingness, Mannion argues that Schopenhauer's philosophy takes a religious turn, concluding that "'behind' the will, there must be 'something' in accord with suggestions of the 'good' and therefore something analogous to theistic interpretations of ultimate reality and the ground of existence."[105] In other words: since Schopenhauer has such a negative understanding of the Will as blind striving flowing through living beings and torturing them relentlessly, this Will *cannot* be the same world-in-itself we become one with through an escape *from* that Will. This interpretation is affirmed by the following observation made by Schopenhauer himself: 'behind our existence lies something else that becomes accessible to us only by our shaking off the world.'[106]

Salvation should, according to this interpretation, be understood as following from a religious revelation, from a 'flash of light' that enlightens one's existence as a suffering individual and that forms a sudden and unexpected 'twist' of knowledge that allows one to experience something hitherto thought impossible. Schopenhauer indeed refers to the notion of 'grace' in this way: 'in consequence of such an effect of grace, man's whole inner nature is fundamentally changed and reversed, so that he no longer wills anything of all that he previously willed so intensely; thus a new man, so to speak, actually takes place of the old.'[107]

Although Mannion hereby seeks to do justice to several important aspects of Schopenhauer's philosophy, I am not convinced by his interpretation. Arguing that we should understand Schopenhauer along religious lines merely removes his theory from the philosophical realm and makes it more speculative by claiming that we have to accept paradoxes as paradoxes, like the religious believer (according to this interpretation) should accept the paradoxes that constitute his or her faith. Mannion's solution furthermore adds an utterly speculative domain to

Schopenhauer's philosophy – a 'benevolent whole' *beyond* the world – and thereby merely corrodes its consistency instead of solidifying it.

Mannion's reading also conflicts with Schopenhauer's ambiguous, and in places, negative, stance towards religion. He often speaks of the hypocritical character of religious persons[108] and proclaims 'all religion' to be 'antagonistic to culture',[109] concluding his essay 'On Religion' as follows:

> In previous centuries religion was a forest behind which armies could halt and take cover. The attempt to repeat this in our day has met with a sharp rebuff. For after so many fellings, it is now only scrub and brushwood, behind which rogues and swindlers occasionally hide themselves. We should, therefore, beware of those who would like to drag it into everything.[110]

Furthermore, at many places Schopenhauer explicitly expresses a fundamental disdain for those religions that deem the world to be 'good', to be created by a benevolent being in the service of human beings. In 'Additional Remarks on the Doctrine of the Suffering in the World' he even explicitly states the following about Leibniz' statement that this is the best of all possible worlds:

> Generally, such a view of the world as the successful work of an all-wise, all-benevolent, and moreover almighty Being is too flagrantly contradicted by the misery and wretchedness that fill the world on the one hand, and by the obvious imperfection and even burlesque distortion of the most perfect of its phenomena on the other; I refer to the human phenomenon. Here is to be found a dissonance that can never be resolved.[111]

We should, however, be careful not to understand these observations too easily as a categorical dismissal of everything religious: Mannion indeed argues that even though Schopenhauer often criticizes overly positive or simplistic forms of religion, his philosophy does contain many positive references to not only Eastern religions, like Buddhism, Hinduism and Sufism, but also to Western ones, especially Christianity. Although Schopenhauer criticizes the idea that there is a personal God and that the universe is created by 'someone' or 'something' for the benefit of human beings, this does not, in other words, mean that his philosophy – especially his idea that we can find peace by becoming one with the essence of the universe – is completely devoid of religious tendencies.[112] At the same time, however, Schopenhauer explicitly claims that he merely refers to the 'allegorical truth'[113] of religious stories and symbols, their being illustrations of a deep metaphysical *need for escape* that does not necessarily imply that there *is* a benevolent 'beyond' that satisfies it.

Conclusion

With an analysis of the notion of salvation, we have arrived at the end of my discussion of Schopenhauer's philosophy. We have seen that Schopenhauer's understanding of this experience is filled with paradoxes and contradictions. Furthermore, he claims that it cannot be put into words, ending his philosophy in a non-conceptual vacuum. Because his mystical observations are surrounded by vagueness, it remains unclear what he precisely means by the process of self-denial. Furthermore, this vagueness results in the fact that different interpretations of his thought have been developed, each following from an aspect of his philosophy: we can read Schopenhauer as developing a fundamental resistance against a world in which suffering takes place, thereby attacking identitarian philosophies and inspiring artists; as constructing a Kierkegaardian view of stages on life's way that results in therapeutic suggestions on how to overcome our condition as suffering beings; or as a religious thinker who eventually claims that a benevolent whole lies behind everything that exists. Even though I have argued that these readings emphasize interesting aspects of his thought but are each too limited and one-sided to be convincing, the fact that his philosophy sparks these different interpretations reflects the unclear nature of his theory of salvation.

Another critical observation is that Schopenhauer's ideas on salvation continue in the same ahistorical vein as the rest of his thought. Happiness or peace cannot be found in social change, in a society that is organized fairly and justly or in a culture that revolves around respect and equality, he suggests. According to Schopenhauer, it lies in a complete turning away from the way of the world, from culture, society and history. Furthermore, he claims that freedom is only found in complete passivity. We only achieve piece, in other words, once we have passively overcome everything that we are and have thrown ourselves into ahistorical nothingness.

In spite of this critique, I want to conclude that Schopenhauer's theory of salvation presents us with several interesting insights. Not only does he develop a philosophy in which the arts play an immensely important role, I also value his idea that the subject has to renounce its dominating and hostile tendencies in order to find peace. This suggests that human beings have to change themselves on a fundamental level in order to better themselves. They have to pierce through the *principium individuationis*, to overcome their tendency to approach everything and everyone only in relation to their own desires, and to elevate themselves to a point of view from which people are not perceived as distinct and separate beings that are each responsible for their own survival. And even though Schopenhauer's mystical turn may be overly radical and rather unconvincing, it does emphasize the idea that this change is extremely difficult.

A last important observation is that Schopenhauer's pessimistic philosophy paradoxically provides us with hope. I herewith follow Horkheimer, who ends his essay 'Schopenhauer today' as follows: 'There are few ideas that the world today needs more than Schopenhauer's – ideas which in the face of utter hopelessness, because they confront it, know more than any others of hope.'[114] Hope is sparked by the observation that one of the bleakest pessimists in the history of philosophy, whose thought revolves around the necessity of suffering and the unfreedom of human beings, eventually arrives at the idea that a change may take place that results in an experience of profound peace. And however unrealistic and vague this ideal may be, its focus on an overcoming of the violent tendencies of the self presents us with a highly critical notion of what such an experience may entail.

10
Rien Faire Comme une Bête

Introduction

In Marcel Proust's *In Search of Lost Time*, most importantly in the second part of its first volume entitled *Swann's Way*, a piano and violin sonata written by the fictitious composer Vinteuil recurs several times. The sonata, which is played at the house of the Verdurin family, contains a melody that Charles Swann associates with his love for Odette and with the experience of happiness. Especially one recurring phrase in the sonata represents a promise of happiness for Swann, a feeling of love that he links to the experience of escaping the immanence of his subjectivity and of opening himself up towards the world. The sonata's effect on Swann is described as follows:

> With a slow and rhythmical movement it led him first this way, then that, towards a state of happiness that was noble, unintelligible, and yet precise. And then suddenly, having reached a certain point from which he was preparing to follow it, after a momentary pause, abruptly it changed direction, and in a fresh movement, more rapid, fragile, melancholy, incessant, sweet, it bore him off with it towards new vistas. Then it vanished. He hoped, with a passionate longing, that he might find it again, a third time. And reappear it did, though without speaking to him more clearly, bringing him, indeed, a pleasure less profound. But when he returned home he felt the need of it: he was like a man into whose life a woman he has seen for a moment passing by has brought the image of a new beauty which deepens his own sensibility, although he does not even know her name or whether he will ever see her again. Indeed this passion for

a phrase of music seemed, for a time, to open up before Swann the possibility of a sort of rejuvenation.[1]

When the love between Swann and Odette starts fading away, the power that the melody holds over Swann only increases; it now represents his longing for an experience of happiness that remains ungraspable, and is described as follows: 'It rippled past, simple and immortal, scattering on every side the bounties of its grace, with the same ineffable smile; but Swann thought that he could now discern in it some disenchantment. It seemed to be aware how vain, how hollow was the happiness to which it showed the way.'[2]

The melody is understood as both expressing the nature of Swann's love – Swann understands the succession of its notes and the crescendo it builds up to as similar to his feelings for Odette – and as representing the ungraspability of happiness, which he experiences as overwhelming and as escaping his self-control. It is described as recalling a 'specific, volatile essence of that lost happiness'[3] and as containing 'forgotten strains of happiness'.[4]

This promise of an ungraspable and unreachable happiness is mirrored in Proust's novel by the happiness that the Narrator finds promised by the names of villages he wanted to visit as a child. In the chapters 'Place-names: the name' (in *Swann's Way*) and 'Place-names: the place' (in *Within a Budding Grove*), Proust describes how, in the mind of a child, the names of places not yet visited are surrounded by a metaphysical aura. This aura triggers expectations and longings in a child's mind and embodies a promise of something ungraspable that is not felt when the place itself is actually visited. The Narrator describes the dreams he has woven around place-names as follows:

> I need only, to make them reappear, pronounce the names Balbec, Venice, Florence, within whose syllables had gradually accumulated the longing inspired in me by the places for which they stood.... But if these names thus permanently absorbed the image I had formed of these towns, it was only by transforming that image, by subordinating its reappearance in me to their own special laws; and in consequence of this they made it more beautiful, but at the same time more different from anything that the towns of Normandy or Tuscany could in reality be, and, by increasing the arbitrary delights of my imagination, aggravated the disenchantment that was in store for me when I set out upon my travels.[5]

In *In Search of Lost Time* happiness is mainly longed-for and not experienced itself. It lies in an ungraspable beyond that is largely based on dreams and expectations that arise in the self and provide the world with an ungraspable aura of promise and hope.

The possibility of metaphysics

In this chapter I will discuss the metaphysical traces that are present in Adorno's philosophy. Apart from Samuel Beckett, I will show that Adorno mentions Proust's writings the most as providing us with models of metaphysical experience.

As in the philosophy of Schopenhauer, Adorno's references to experiences of a metaphysical nature have to be understood against the background of an almost inescapable whole that imprisons the subject and that, as we have seen in Chapters 5, 6 and 8, makes it almost impossible to refer to experiences of a positive nature. As I have argued in the case of Schopenhauer, this means, first and foremost, that Adorno's metaphysics cannot and should not affirm the whole that we are part of as fundamentally good or benevolent. Metaphysical experiences therefore partly revolve, in Adorno's view, around a resistance against historical conditions that cause suffering:

> In the face of the experiences we have had, not only through Auschwitz but through the introduction of torture as a permanent institution and through the atomic bomb – all these things form a kind of coherence, a hellish unity – in the face of these experiences the assertion that what is has meaning, and the affirmative character which has been attributed to metaphysics almost without exception, become a mockery; and in the face of the victims it becomes downright immoral.[6]

Unlike Schopenhauer's thought, Adorno's philosophy only contains sporadic references to experiences that he characterizes as 'metaphysical'. In this sense, his discussion of metaphysics follows his analysis of morality: whereas Schopenhauer explicitly describes compassion and develops a theory about moral and anti-moral incentives, Adorno refers to rather ungraspable physical impulses. Concerning the realm of metaphysics, his descriptions are equally fragmentary and vague.

This is a direct result of the observation that, from a certain perspective, Adorno's thought is more negative than Schopenhauer's: even though the latter frequently refers to slavery, torture and war and does not hesitate to call the world a manifestation of evil, his pessimism is characterized by an innocence that Adorno's theory lacks, constituted as it is 'after Auschwitz'. Even though Adorno's metaphysical observations follow the negative nature of Schopenhauer's, in other words, they go one step further. In his lectures on *Metaphysics* Adorno describes this difference as follows:

> Schopenhauer ... was a pessimist ... and vehemently opposed the affirmative character of metaphysics .... Nevertheless, in his work he turned even this negativity into a metaphysical principle, the principle of the blind will which, because it is a metaphysical principle and therefore a category of reflection, contains the possibility of its own negation by human beings. Thus, he also posits the idea of the denial of the Will to Live, a denial which, in view of what has been and continues to be perpetrated on the living and can increase to an unimaginable degree, is an almost comforting idea. I mean that in a world which knows of things far worse than death and denies people the shot in the neck in order to torture them slowly to death, the doctrine of the denial of the Will to Live itself has something of the innocence for which Schopenhauer criticized the theodicies of philosophers.[7]

The bleakness, the hopelessness and the anxiety caused by an almost complete destruction of meaning are, in other words, described by Adorno as having such a 'compelling universality'[8] or 'hellish unity'[9] – such a gruesome and all-permeating inescapability that even Schopenhauer's radical theory of salvation is characterized as naïve.

In his 'Meditations on Metaphysics', which close *Negative Dialectics*, Adorno keeps returning, however, to the question of whether metaphysical experience is still possible in a world after Auschwitz, in a culture that he describes, with reference to Brecht, as 'built of dogshit'.[10] These meditations circle around two problems. First, Adorno describes the incapacity of the modern subject to experience any kind of metaphysical transcendence, arguing that 'our metaphysical faculty is paralyzed because actual events have shattered the basis on which speculative metaphysical thought could be reconciled with experience'.[11] In places, he even seems to equate metaphysical experience with experience *itself*, arguing that the world in which we live is so overwhelmingly distorted and reified that experience has become metaphysical in nature. Indeed, he describes the doctrine of empiricism as containing a metaphysical moment: 'empiricism, with its emphasis on empirical sources, implies an element of metaphysics at least in the sense that the essential knowledge is seen as that which does not coincide with concepts, but which, as it were, falls accidentally into my lap, and thus always includes the possibility that it might not do so.'[12]

Second, Adorno claims that even if it were possible to have a transcending experience and feel at home in the world, this would be morally wrong: 'After Auschwitz, our feelings resist any claim of the positivity of existence as sanctimonious, as wronging the victims; they balk at squeezing any kind of sense, however bleached, out of the victims' fate.'[13]

Like a pendulum, however, the 'Meditations on Metaphysics' swing back and forth between claims regarding the impossibility of metaphysical experience on the one hand, and a yearning for these kinds of experiences on the other. Even though he deems metaphysics to be impossible, Adorno paradoxically argues that it is only in metaphysical experiences that we can place hope. These experiences are our only chance at getting a glimpse of something different, a glimpse of otherness.

The mechanisms underlying his attempts to develop an understanding of the metaphysical in a world in which this seems impossible can best be illustrated by quoting a lengthy passage in which Adorno, again, discusses Schopenhauer's ideas on the denial of the Will:

> As a positive statement, the thesis that life is senseless would be as foolish as it is false to avow the contrary; the thesis is true only as a blow at the high-flown avowal. Nor is Schopenhauer's inclination to identify the essence of the world, the blind will, as absolutely negative from a human viewpoint any longer fitting. The claim of total subsumption is far too analogous to the positive claim of Schopenhauer's despised contemporaries, the idealists.... Compared with Schopenhauer's irrationalism, the monotheism he attacked in a spirit of enlightenment has some truth to it also. Schopenhauer's metaphysics regresses to a phase before the awakening of genius amidst the mute world. He denies the motive of freedom, the motive men remember for the time being and even, perhaps, in the phase of total unfreedom. Schopenhauer gets to the bottom of the delusiveness of individuation, but his recipe for freedom in Book Four, to deny the will to live, is no less delusive – as if the ephemerally individualized could have the slightest power over its negative absolute, the will as a thing in itself; as if it could escape from the spell of that will without either deceiving itself or allowing the whole metaphysics of the will to get away through the gap. Total determinism is no less mythical than

> are the totalities of Hegel's logic. Schopenhauer was an idealist *malgré lui-même*, a spokesman of the spell. The *totum* is the totem. Grayness could not fill us with despair if our minds did not harbour the concept of different colors, scattered traces of which are not absent from the negative whole. The traces always come from the past, and our hopes come from their counterpart, from that which was or is doomed.[14]

Adorno here criticizes the paradox that underlies Schopenhauer's theory of salvation, following from the latter's idea that we can deny everything that we are by *wilfully* exterminating the Will. But Adorno also criticizes the totalizing nature of Schopenhauer's bleak conclusions: like Hegel, he argues, Schopenhauer merely projects a conceptual idea onto the world as a whole. And whether this idea is 'Will' or 'Spirit', negative or positive in nature, its character is idealistic since it overlooks the particularities of the world, the 'different colors' that form the (positive) framework within we are able to understand our experiences of a world defined by Will as negative and 'grey'.[15]

Adorno furthermore follows Lukács, writing that even though Schopenhauer's ideas on the Will reflect the unfreedom of the modern individual, they merely affirm the inescapability of this unfreedom by claiming that the historical situation they reflect follows from the way the world essentially is. Thereby, Schopenhauer denies what Adorno calls the 'motive of freedom', which may still be present in the minds of a few precisely because the world has not always been like it is and does not always have to be like this.

Following this critique, Adorno argues that metaphysical experiences are short, sporadic, ungraspable and vulnerable in nature. They exist in the cracks of a whole that Schopenhauer, in Adorno's view, too easily identifies as completely determined: 'micrology is the place where metaphysics finds a haven from totality.'[16]

And whereas Schopenhauer places these experiences in a 'beyond', in a radical turning away from what he ahistorically defines as an illusory and false existence, Adorno's observations on the social nature of this engulfing whole allow him to argue that metaphysical experiences can be found in moments in which this false whole is partly transcended. Whereas Schopenhauer, furthermore, refers to experiences that are timeless and ahistorical, Adorno places hope in personal moments that are constituted in specific places and have a specific and individual nature and history, like the ungraspable aura that, in Swann's experience, surrounds Vinteuil's sonata.[17] In the following, I want to discuss two of the experiences Adorno refers to in the context of metaphysics.

Happiness and peace

Childhood memories

In his lectures on *Metaphysics* Adorno discusses Marcel Proust and touches on the first definition of metaphysical experiences that I want to analyse. Not only does he feel an affinity with the 'micrological' and extremely personal nature of Proust's descriptions in *In Search of Lost Time*, he is specifically interested in the understanding of happiness that he distils from Proust's masterwork, arguing that 'there is an extremely deep constellation between metaphysical experience and happiness'.[18]

To highlight the metaphysical nature of these experiences, Adorno refers to the above-discussed promise of happiness embodied, in Proust's writings, by the names of villages one visited as a child. Adorno discusses these observations as follows in relation to his own personal experiences with villages in Germany: 'When one is on holiday as a child and reads or hears names like Monbrunn, Reuenthal, Hambrunn, one has the feeling: if only one were there, at that place, that would be it. This "it" – what the "it" is – is extraordinarily difficult to say; one will probably be able to say, following Proust's tracks here too, that it is happiness.'[19]

Adorno characterizes this happiness as metaphysical because the experience promised by the village name is vulnerable, fleeting and ungraspable.[20] Being in the village, one has the feeling that one is too close to it to actually be happy, to grasp the happiness that the village embodies from a distance. He illustrates the ungraspability of this promise of happiness with the image of a rainbow[21] and argues that 'the person who is happy is too close to this "it" to be able to have any standpoint towards it within consciousness'.[22]

These observations highlight two characteristics of Adorno's understanding of metaphysical experiences. First, they are what he calls 'fallible' in nature.[23] Like the promise of happiness recalled by village names, or like a *déjà vu* 'induced by a certain type of children's book',[24] they are constituted by a combination of one's longings, remembrances, hopes and desires on the one hand, and an opening up towards the world on the other. Since this world can fail to conform to one's memories or desires – the village we visit can fail to make us happy – metaphysical experiences follow from the attempt to grasp a receding reality; an ungraspable and vulnerable otherness.

The second aspect of these experiences consists of what Adorno famously dubs the 'preponderance of the object'. He herewith refers to a contact with the objective world – constituting what he calls an 'objective moment'[25] – that makes room for the element of surprise and, again, fallibility. The subject opens itself in these experiences up towards the world, submits its longings, needs and desires to it and thereby constitutes the above-discussed possibility of failure. In an insightful passage, Proust describes the ungraspability and fallibility Adorno refers to as follows:

> When I saw an external object, my consciousness that I was seeing it would remain between me and it, surrounding it with a thin spiritual border that prevented me from ever touching its substance directly; for it would somehow evaporate before I could make contact with it, just as an incandescent body that is brought into proximity with something wet never actually touches its moisture, since it is always preceded by a zone of evaporation.[26]

What characterizes these metaphysical experiences furthermore is that they have to be *lived*, in Adorno's view: like a child, one has to be embedded in the world, carefree, as it were, entrusting oneself to a whole that is seemingly endless and contains the possibility of surprise, unexpectedness and happiness at its horizon. Again, Proust's highly detailed descriptions of smell, light and colour come to mind as sensory forms of contact with a world that is 'open'. Like Schopenhauer, Adorno here seeks refuge in almost mystical formulations that, in their vagueness, refer to an experience of life that cannot be put into words: 'nothing can be even experienced as living if it does not contain a promise of something transcending life. This transcendence therefore is, and at the same time is not – and beyond that contradiction it is no doubt very difficult, and probably impossible, for thought to go.'[27]

The impossibility of happiness

It is important to notice that Adorno refers to childhood experiences in this context – to an experience of transcendence, in other words, that took place in the past and that may have provided us with an experience of otherness that sheds light on the wrongness of the status quo.[28] This again forces us to address the question around which his 'Meditations on Metaphysics' revolve: is it possible to have experiences of a metaphysical nature in the here and now? In a whole that is false, the only experience of transcendence, Adorno seems to argue, can be found in a remembrance of playfulness and naïve happiness that contrasts dramatically with the status quo.

Not coincidentally we find a similar contrast between a happy childhood and a false present in the second volume of Schopenhauer's *The World as Will and Representation*: 'childhood is the time of innocence and happiness, the paradise of life, the lost Eden, on which we look back longingly through the whole remaining course of our life.'[29] But whereas Schopenhauer, of course, argues that this childhood happiness *always* gets overshadowed by an overpowering and tormenting Will – in fact, he describes puberty as the tragic end of childhood happiness, since sexual urges then start to torment the individual – Adorno claims that the distorting nature of our *specific* time and age makes childhood happiness and its naive openness towards the world into an exemplary remembrance of transcendence.

It has been argued that sexual love can be understood as containing, at least, a promise of the kind of happiness Adorno describes with reference to Proust.[30] According to this reading, sexual pleasure allows one to break through one's immanence and connect to another being in a way that is not mediated by falseness. The vulnerability displayed in sexual love and the openness towards the other person, in other words, constitute an experience of transcendence that, within Adorno's grim understanding of the imprisoned subject, could be understood as metaphysical in nature.

These hedonistic ideas, revolving around a longing for experiences of fulfilment that cannot really be put into words,[31] however, conflict acutely with the otherwise grave negativity of Adorno's thought. This is especially the case since, as we have seen in Chapter 5, Adorno describes sexual pleasure and bodily experiences as permeated and distorted by the culture industry, providing a 'false' catharsis.[32] In *Aesthetic Theory*, furthermore, Adorno explicitly states that the culture industry 'plans for and exploits the need for happiness'[33] and that 'all happiness found in the status quo is an ersatz and false'.[34]

In the text following his above-cited lengthy analysis of Schopenhauer's denial of Will, Adorno furthermore praises the 'incomparable power' of 'Proust the metaphysicist' because he tried, 'with the unbridled urge to happiness', to look for sense and meaning in the experience of 'fulfilled moments'.[35] Even Proust, however, eventually had to conclude that happiness cannot be found in the idea of the 'fullness of life', Adorno observes, because his understanding of this experience is overshadowed in his novel by death: 'Since death is irrevocable, it is ideological to assert that a meaning might rise in the light of fragmentary, albeit genuine, experience. This is why one of the central points of his work, the death of Bergotte, finds Proust helping, gropingly, to express hope for a resurrection – against all the philosophy of life, yet without seeking cover from the positive religions.'[36] Following his interpretation of Proust, Adorno therefore argues that it is not 'in the moments of present existence'[37] that happiness should be sought, but in a resistance against the grim nature of an existence that undermines the possibility of happiness.

Peace

Adorno partly contradicts himself, however: his works contain references to an experience that comes close to a happiness found in the here and now. In an aphorism in *Minima Moralia* called 'Sur L'Eau' – named after the title of book sketches on sailing by Maupassant[38] – Adorno describes this experience as follows:

> *Rien faire comme une bête*, lying on water and looking peacefully at the sky, 'being, nothing else, without any definition and fulfilment', might take the place of process, act, satisfaction, and so truly keep the promise of dialectical logic that it would culminate in its origin. None of the abstract concepts comes closer to fulfilled utopia than that of eternal peace.[39]

The experience described here is not coincidental or brief in nature. Unlike the promise of childhood happiness, furthermore, it is not based on expectancies, needs and longings that one 'submits' to the objective world. And unlike sexual pleasure, this experience is not aimed at active gratification or satisfaction.

At the same time, however, this experience is profoundly corporeal: whereas Adorno, as we have seen in Chapter 8, defines his ethics as consisting of the attempt to 'be a good animal', the animality of our embodied existence returns in the above-quoted definition of peace. The purposelessness, naivety and innocence that characterize the lives of animals provide us with an example of an existence that is different from the life we lead as mere instruments of a social condition. The nothingness of animal existence, the 'bliss', to put it in Schopenhauer's terms, of an existence that is not permeated with reified categories, nor by a gap between self and body or subject and object, shows us a specific manner of being that is radically different from a world defined by domination. In *Minima Moralia* Adorno observes in this context, referring to Marx's analysis of commodification described in Chapter 5:

> The relation of children to animals depends entirely on the fact that Utopia goes disguised in creatures whom Marx even begrudged the surplus value they contribute as workers. In existing without any

> purpose recognizable to men, animals hold out, as if for expression, their own names, utterly impossible to exchange. This makes them so beloved to children, their contemplation so blissful.[40]

It is important to emphasize that these descriptions contain an ungraspable, even utopian element: they are references to an experience that might come close to peace, but it remains unclear if having such an experience is actually possible in the status quo. This uncertainty and ungraspability is insightfully put into words by Proust in a passage in which he describes the river Vivonne. This passage might have influenced Adorno's reference to lying on one's back on water:

> How often have I watched, and longed to imitate when I should be free to live as I chose, a rower who had shipped his oars and lay flat on his back in the bottom of his boat, letting it drift with the current, seeing nothing but the sky gliding slowly by above him, his face aglow with a foretaste of happiness and peace![41]

I want to shed light on the nature of this experience by looking at Adorno's observations on boredom in the aphorism 'Spoilsport' in *Minima Moralia*. In this aphorism Adorno refers to Schopenhauer's claim that we feel bored when our desires and needs are for a brief moment satisfied, because we then experience 'an empty longing for a new desire'.[42] The overpowering whole that, in Schopenhauer's view, defines our lives as striving and desiring creatures – Will – defines our existence even when we do not actively strive for satisfaction. Adorno historicizes this observation by claiming that even a respite from labour – free time – is permeated with bourgeois categories:

> [Schopenhauer's] concept of boredom, raised to such unsuspected dignity, is – and this is the last thing that Schopenhauer's anti-historical mind would admit – bourgeois through and through. It is the complement of alienated labour, being the experience of antithetically 'free time', whether because this latter is intended only to restore the energy expended, or because the appropriation of alien labour weighs on it like a mortgage. Free time remains the reflex-action to a production rhythm imposed heteronomously on the subject, compulsively maintained even in the weary pauses. Consciousness of the unfreedom of existence in its entirety, suppressed by the demands of earning a living, that is, by unfreedom itself, only emerges in the intermezzo of freedom.[43]

In his essay 'Free Time', in which he returns to Schopenhauer's ideas on boredom,[44] Adorno again observes that 'free time depends on the totality of social conditions, which continues to hold people under its spell. Neither in their work nor in their consciousness do people dispose of genuine freedom'.[45]

Whereas Schopenhauer argues that a short respite from the Will can only be experienced as mediated by Will and therefore results in boredom, Adorno observes that free time can only be experienced as mediated by the social conditions from which one claims to be free: we feel bored because we feel that we should do something with our free time, because the experience of freedom is permeated with the notions of efficiency and productivity and is therefore essentially unfreedom.

Like Schopenhauer, Adorno seeks to escape from the overpowering influence of this false whole by way of a metaphysical experience of blissful nothingness, which he describes in the above-cited passage on peace. In contrast with 'free time', this experience is defined not by 'acting' or by striving for 'satisfaction', nor by boredom or 'empty restlessness', but by an animalistic nothingness in which one nevertheless feels completely at ease, liquefying the boundaries between oneself and one's environment, and oneself and one's body, in an almost mystical awareness of animalistic being.

A stratum of mute reference to what is beautiful

Like Schopenhauer, Adorno not only discusses experiences he characterizes as metaphysical in nature, he also places hope in the realm of aesthetics and in the ability of artworks to constitute a metaphysical moment. Since the scope of this book does not allow me to discuss Adorno's complex aesthetic theory as a whole, I want to focus on two aspects of his ideas on art and metaphysics that allow me to contrast his ideas with Schopenhauer's: tragic art and, again, a longing for peace.

Form, Absurdity, Distortion

The first aspect of Adorno's aesthetic theory brings us again to Samuel Beckett, especially to his play *Endgame*. In his article on Beckett and Schopenhauer, cited in Chapter 9, Gottfried Büttner mentions how Schopenhauer's understanding of tragic art had an important influence on Beckett's writings, especially mentioning Beckett's Schopenhauerian claim that tragic plays reflect the 'original sin' that consists of being born.[46] Adorno, in turn, notices in his dense essay on *Endgame* that the play expresses a Schopenhauerian negation of the will to life[47] and states in his lectures on *Metaphysics* that the dramas of Beckett are the 'only truly relevant metaphysical productions since the war', as mentioned in Chapter 5.[48]

With this latter observation, he refers firstly to the Schopenhauerian idea, following from the latter's observations on tragedy, that artworks – in this case Beckett's dramas – mimic the falseness of a whole that individuals find themselves embedded in. Whereas Schopenhauer, however, argues that this whole consists of the engulfing nature of Will, diminishing the autonomy and freedom of the tragic hero, Adorno claims that this falseness corrupts the self on an even more fundamental level. He argues that the self has lost its grip on the world completely and has disintegrated into the powerless state that Beckett's play describes, a state in which even words and concepts have lost their meaning.

Endgame depicts a world in which subjectivity has dissolved and in which life has been reduced to mere survival: the world has no meaning anymore, since the subject is too damaged to know what meaning is or what it can cling to in order to find a sense of belonging or unity.[49] Beckett himself indeed observed: 'It's not even possible to talk about truth. That's part of the anguish.'[50] In the last pages of his essay on *Endgame*, Adorno puts this idea into words as follows, referring to the above-mentioned death of Bergotte in Proust's *In Search of Lost Time*:

> Consciousness gets ready to look its own end in the eye, as though it wanted to survive in the way these two [CLOV and HAMM, protagonists of *Endgame*] have survived the destruction of their world. Proust, about whom Beckett wrote an essay in his youth, is said to have tried to record his own death throes; the notes were to be inserted into the description of Bergotte's death. *Endgame* carries out this intention as though it were a mandate bequeathed in a will.[51]

Whereas Schopenhauer argues that the manner in which tragic plays mimic reality provides its spectators with insight into their situation, Adorno describes in *Aesthetic Theory* how *Endgame*'s reflection of meaninglessness forces its readers to realize something about the nature of their world as well, pushing 'its situation so far that it becomes the critique of this situation':[52]

> Beckett's oeuvre already presupposes [the] experience of the destruction of meaning as self-evident, yet also pushes it beyond meaning's abstract negation in that his plays force the traditional categories of art to undergo this experience... Beckett's plays are absurd not

> because of the absence of any meaning, for then they would be simply irrelevant, but because they put meaning on trial; they unfold its history.[53]

The difference between Schopenhauer and Adorno's understandings of metaphysical experience translates itself here into the difference between their analyses of what art does and can do. Whereas Schopenhauer, writing 'before Auschwitz', could still claim that tragic artworks 'represent' the powerlessness of the subject, Adorno argues that the permeation of thought and experience with wrong social categories is so extreme that the explicit conceptualization of the individual's unfreedom is not possible anymore: subjects have lost the freedom necessary to develop distance and self-reflection, and do not have the concepts at hand that would enable them to do this – these concepts have been reduced to mere meaningless sounds, like the words uttered by the characters in *Endgame*.[54]

In other words: art cannot escape reality and constitute experiences of timelessness, like in Schopenhauer's theory, but has to seek refuge in absurdity and extreme distortion to be able to turn against the false whole that produced it, Adorno observes:

> Art keeps itself alive through its social force of resistance.... Its contribution to society is not communication with it but rather something extremely mediated: It is resistance in which, by virtue of inner-aesthetic development, social development is reproduced without being imitated. At the risk of its self-alienation, radical modernity preserves art's immanence by admitting society only in an obscured form.[55]

Schopenhauer's emphasis on the content of artworks is hereby transformed into a concern with the style and form of art, which both mimics and transgresses the falseness of the culture in which we live. Art, Adorno herewith argues, cannot escape the subject's domination: it is produced, made out of materials, and is therefore still a way of shaping and distorting the object.[56] Nevertheless, it can do this in such a way that it turns these techniques against themselves.

This idea returns in Adorno's analysis of Arnold Schönberg's twelve-tone technique. Being concerned with the way in which the culture industry, in Adorno's view, industrializes and commercializes music, making it into mere entertainment that provides us with standardized and false images of happiness, Adorno praises Schönberg's method for forcing the composer to overcome the traditional tonal system. This not only results in music that refuses to be usurped by the culture industry's commodification or the standardizing tendencies of identity-thinking, it also criticizes these mechanisms by taking them to the extreme: 'Twelve-tone technique is truly the fate of music. It enchains music by liberating it. The subject dominates music through the rationality of the system, only in order to succumb to the rational system itself.'[57]

We have seen in Chapter 8 that Adorno describes a similar procedure in the context of Kafka's narratives about animals, which critically reflect the reduction of the modern subject to an animalistic state: 'Myth is to succumb by its own reflected image.'[58] This concern with style and exaggeration makes Adorno praise other forms of modern art as well, for example Picasso's *Guernica*:

> It can be said that philosophy, and theoretical thought as a whole, suffers from an idealist prejudice insofar as it disposes solely over concepts; only through them does it treat what they are concerned with, which it itself never has. ... Modern art has registered dissatisfaction with this ever since Picasso disrupted his pictures with scraps of newspaper, an act from which all montage derives.[59]

Modern works of art, in other words, are partly able to critically break the power that conceptual thinking has over the subject by creating obscurity, debating the meaning of meaning – like Beckett's absurdist plays – or by reflecting the unclear and distorted nature of the subject's experience: 'The idea that the work of art should manifest observable clarity leads to the illusion that the dichotomy between subject and object has been overcome.'[60]

Metaphysical moments

This brings us to the second aspect of Adorno's aesthetic theory that I want to discuss in this chapter: the manner in which certain works of art, in his view, manage to constitute a metaphysical moment. Again, these experiences revolve within an Adornian context around a crippled and almost completely powerless self that seeks to cling to something outside of itself.

In his lectures on *Metaphysics* Adorno is perhaps the clearest about the nature of this moment. Referring again to Brecht's line that 'humanity up to now has built itself an immense palace of dogshit',[61] he states the following:

> If one realizes that everything we call culture consists in the suppression of nature and any uncontrolled traces of nature, then what this

culture finds most unbearable are those places where it is not quite able to control natural manifestations, where they intrude persistently into its own domain.[62]

Based on this rather totalizing claim, Adorno argues that Beckett's dramas, especially *Endgame*, are metaphysical in nature because they force us to look at a repressed natural manifestation that he describes with phrases that I cited in previous chapters as well: as a 'place of carrion, stench and putrefaction'; a 'dark stratum' that philosophy seeks to repress or ignore; a sphere in which people 'vegetate between life and death – as they actually vegetated in the concentration camps'.[63]

Beckett's play forces us to realize that both philosophy and human connections have been reduced to garbage: 'philosophy, spirit itself, declares itself to be dead inventory, the dreamlike leavings of the world of experience, and the poetic process declares itself to be a process of wastage'[64] and: '*Endgame* prepares us for a state of affairs in which everyone who lifts the lid of the nearest trashcan can expect to find his own parents in it. The natural connection between the living has now become organic garbage.'[65]

This analysis of Beckett's *Endgame* contains traces of Adorno's ideas on morality, referring to 'the moment of aversion to the inflicting of physical pain on what Brecht once called the torturable body of any person'.[66] The social whole that Adorno describes, in other words, has reduced both moral experiences *and* metaphysical experiences to the 'zone of the carcass' referred to in Chapter 8: 'Metaphysics, I say, has slipped into material existence. Precisely this transition of metaphysical questions and, if I might state it so grandly, of metaphysics itself to this stratum of the material, is what is repressed by the conniving consciousness, the official yes-saying of whatever ilk.'[67]

This means that the transcendent and metaphysical moment found in Beckett's play makes this play into a critique of the culture that it mimics: in a whole that is false and that leaves us no escape, any kind of transcendence has a critical edge, confronting us with something that this whole rejects – in this case bodily suffering. In *Negative Dialectics* Adorno therefore returns to his infamous statement that it is barbaric to write poetry after Auschwitz: 'Perennial suffering has as much right to expression as a tortured man has to scream; hence it may have been wrong to say that after Auschwitz you could no longer write poems.'[68]

In this context we may think of the suffering of humans and animals depicted on Picasso's *Guernica*, or the suffering, demonic flesh linked to an anonymous, modern businessman on Francis Bacon's *Painting*

(1964). But Adorno also mentions music in this context. In a passage on Schönberg and Webern, for example, he connects the above-described ability of modern music to mirror the domination on which society rests to the expression of bodily suffering: 'Musical language is polarized according to its extremes: towards gestures of shock resembling bodily convulsions on the one hand, and on the other towards a crystalline standstill of a human being whom anxiety causes to freeze in her tracks.'[69] As in his analysis of Beckett's *Endgame*, Adorno links a domination of form that results in absurdity and ungraspability to the inability of the modern subject to express itself and to the 'twitching' of crippled and suffering bodies.

A broken promise of happiness

These disturbing references to a repressed natural manifestation, bordering on Adorno's analysis of morality, are not the only metaphysical experiences that artworks constitute, according to his analysis. As in the case of the above-described promise of happiness embodied by names of villages one visited as a child, Adorno argues as well that certain artworks recall a longing towards 'something' that is expected by a consciousness reaching out to the world on the one hand, and a world in which this longing never really finds the longed-for object or experience on the other: 'Aesthetic experience is that of something that spirit may find neither in the world nor in itself; it is possibility promised by its impossibility. Art is the ever broken promise of happiness.'[70] Again we herewith arrive at the observation that whereas Schopenhauer could still refer to an experience of happiness found directly in aesthetic contemplation, Adorno provides the subject with even less freedom and almost completely throws it back upon itself, replacing happiness with a broken promise of happiness.[71]

But although Adorno keeps insisting that happiness does not exist anymore in the here and now, he develops an understanding of 'beauty' in which his above-described reference to the experience of peace returns. He writes in a rich passage in *Aesthetic Theory*:

> What is no longer socially possible in traditional art does not on that account surrender all truth. Instead it sinks to a historical, geological stratum that is no longer accessible to consciousness except through negation but without which no art would exist: a stratum of mute reference to what is beautiful, without all that strict a distinction between nature and work. This element is contrary to the disintegrative element into which the truth of art has changed; yet it survives

> because as the forming force it recognizes the violence of that by which it measures itself. It is through this idea that art is related to peace. Without perspective on peace, art would be as untrue as when it anticipates reconciliation. Beauty in art is the semblance of the truly peaceful.[72]

By struggling to represent peace, artworks express the impossibility of this experience in the current world *and* allude to it at the same time. By denying the possibility of catharsis, of satisfaction, of reconciliation, reflecting the objectivity of this impossibility under social conditions, they paradoxically refer to 'the truly peaceful'. It is, in my view, important to notice that Adorno here again refers to a 'stratum', like he does in his analysis of the metaphysical moment of Beckett's *Endgame*. The body, peace, happiness and metaphysics, he implies, have been pushed away by a whole that is false but still 'exists' somewhere in a distorted manner, at the bottom of Beckett's 'corpsed' world. Proust's above-mentioned reference to 'forgotten strains of happiness' comes to mind as well.

Like Schopenhauer, Adorno is most explicit about this experience in his writings on music. The non-conceptual nature of music, he argues, allows it to refer to 'something' without making this 'something' visible. Schönberg's method of composing, for example, not only mirrors and parodies the rational, enlightened subject that imposes its conceptual structures on the world, in his view, but does this so radically that this results in music that refuses to be completely absorbed by this same subject. Hereby this method produces music that rejects traditional forms of meaning and confronts the self with an abstract yet powerful otherness, which contains flashes of a different kind of existence: 'The emancipation of music today is tantamount to its emancipation from verbal language, and it is this emancipation which flashes during the destruction of "meaning".'[73] Music shows us a relationship between subject and object that is radically different from the domination inherent to identity-thinking.

But whereas his analysis of Schönberg mainly focuses on the control exercised by style and form, at other places Adorno expresses an almost Schopenhauerian analysis of that which music might represent: his interpretations of Schönberg's compositions and Beckett's *Endgame* require reflection and conceptual analysis, but his works also contain hints regarding more direct aesthetic experiences. In several passages, Adorno argues that the unique and non-conceptual nature of music enables it to hint at a 'broken' and 'lost' relationship between subject and object that conceptual languages by definition cannot evoke. This nature consists of an absence of egotistic needs and drives and an almost self-less form of contemplation: 'music moves towards the pure name, the absolute unity of thing and sign, which is lost in its immediacy to all human knowledge.'[74]

This almost hidden aspect of Adorno's thoughts on music is noticed by Espen Hammer, who observes about Adorno's essay on Schubert: 'deeply buried in the semantic layer of Adorno's materialism there is a Schopenhauerian longing not only for an unguarded encounter with the not-I, but a submersion into an unmasterable, Dionysian alterity, culminating in the complete indistinction between subject and object.'[75] Indeed, Adorno writes rather uncharacteristically in this essay about the 'holes in the foreground of form' that Schubert's themes appear as, providing us with glimpses of an 'unattainable true form'.[76] He also refers to Schubert's 'landscape of death', in which Schubert's themes stand 'timelessly side by side', filling 'a rediscovered time far from the finality of death with the anticipated permanence of the Eternal'.[77]

In *Philosophy of Modern Music* we find another rather uncharacteristic reference to this aspect of music. Adorno there not only quotes Goethe and refers to a 'return to the earth', he also stresses that the expression of music contains a bodily – almost primitive – dimension, irreducible to subjectivity or intentionality, which allows the subject to 'enter into alienated territory':

> Music and tears open the lips and set the arrested human being free. The sentimentality of inferior music indicates in its distorted figure that which higher music, at the very border of insanity, is yet able to design in the validity of its form: reconciliation. The human being who surrenders himself to tears and to a music which no longer resembles him in any way permits that current of which he is not part and which lies behind the dam restraining the world of phenomena to flow back into itself. In weeping and in singing he enters into alienated reality. 'Tears dim my eyes: earth's child I am again' – this line from Goethe's *Faust* defines the position of music. Thus earth claims Eurydice again. The gesture of return – not the sensation of expectancy – characterizes the expression of all music, even if it finds itself in a world worthy of death.[78]

The experience here described comes close to Adorno's above-cited references to peace, to an almost animalistic 'return' to and embeddedness in the world. The peace that is present, as a 'mute stratum', in musical compositions, consists of a calming down of one's otherwise hostile and conceptual approach to the world. It revolves around the constitution of a stance of respect and openness towards otherness and an overcoming of feelings of aggressiveness, domination and control.

Like Schopenhauer, Adorno herewith argues that the main difference between aesthetic experiences and 'regular' experiences is found in the way in which the subject relates to the object: instead of perceiving everything in relation to a violent drive to self-preservation, aesthetic experiences are based on the subject's openness and trust. In *Aesthetic Theory* Adorno indeed refers to Schopenhauer to illustrate this idea: 'aesthetic experience, as Schopenhauer knew, breaks through the spell of obstinate self-preservation; it is the model of a stage of consciousness in which the I no longer has its happiness in its interests, or, ultimately, in its reproduction.'[79]

Social change

A good society

In one of the last pages of 'Meditations on Metaphysics', Adorno returns to Schopenhauer again and discusses the latter's claim that 'the world is just a hell and in it human beings are the tortured souls on the one hand, and the devils on the other':[80]

> The world is worse than hell, and it is better. It is worse, because even nihility could not be that absolute as which it finally appears conciliatory in Schopenhauer's Nirvana. There is no way out of the closed context of immanence; it denies the world even the measure of sense accorded to it by the Hindu philosopheme that views it as the dream of an evil demon. The mistake in Schopenhauer's thinking is that the law which keeps immanence under its own spell is directly said to be that essence which immanence blocks, the essence that would not be conceivable as other than transcendent. But the world is better than hell because the absolute conclusiveness which Schopenhauer attributes to the world's course is borrowed in turn from the idealistic system.[81]

Again, Adorno here criticizes Schopenhauer's metaphysics of Will for being as totalizing as Hegel's idealism. But in this passage he not only uses this critique to argue that metaphysical experiences are possible in the here and now, but also to refer to the necessity of social change.

Schopenhauer is too optimistic, Adorno argues, since his theory of salvation provides us with a rather clear method of escape, with a way out provided by a metaphysical system that allows us to shake off the world completely if we let go of the illusory 'veil' the subject projects upon this world. Since this 'veil' is a concept, an abstraction, Adorno argues, it can be easily thought of as 'something' that can disappear. Schopenhauer's philosophy is too pessimistic, on the other hand, because it closes the door completely to any change in a here and now that is understood as essentially driven by an unchangeable metaphysical core.

This brings us to the last aspect of Adorno's thought that I want to discuss. Whereas he argues that the above-described metaphysical experiences are momentary in nature, consisting of flashes and glimpses, true happiness and long-lasting peace can only be found in a society in which unnecessary suffering is no more, his philosophy suggests.

It is impossible, however, to develop a clear idea of what a good society looks like in a whole that is false, just like – as we have seen in Chapter 8 – it is impossible to refer to a notion of the good life in a world in which no real living takes place. In *Capital* Marx states about the coming about of a better society: 'The whole mystery of commodities, all the magic and necromancy that surrounds the products of labour on the basis of commodity production, vanishes ... as soon as we come to other forms of production.'[82] Adorno refers to this passage in *Negative Dialectics*: 'A change in the conditions of production might relieve the violent picture which the world shows to its violators.'[83] The constitution of a better society is only possible, in other words, once people become aware of the actual unfreedom in which they live.[84]

We have seen, however, that Adorno claims that a system has come into being that permeates people's thoughts, ideas and experiences and that makes the social conditions under which they live appear as necessary; as second nature. Furthermore, he argues that all-present and all-dominating institutions like the culture industry create such a wrong picture of the world that most people are guided by created needs and false notions of happiness and freedom. It therefore becomes very difficult for him to argue that the veil covering social relations can be removed or pierced through at all.

If we can speak of Adornian descriptions of a good society, these are therefore mostly negative in nature, consisting of a radical rejection of the status quo. One cannot, in other words, distil a social and political normative theory from his thought as systematic and detailed as developed by thinkers belonging to later generations of the Frankfurt

School – most obvious examples are, of course, Jürgen Habermas' *Theory of Communicative Action* and Axel Honneth's *The Struggle for Recognition*.[85] In places, Adorno indeed characterizes the idea of a good society as utopian in nature, deliberately keeping it vague and out of reach. He refers, for example, to 'the Utopia that once drew sustenance from motherly love'[86] and in the above-described aphorism 'Sur L'Eau' he refers to 'eternal peace' as 'fulfilled utopia'.[87]

Nevertheless, Adorno's philosophy contains glimpses of what a good society may look like. Following his reference to Marx cited above, for example, he argues that the construction of such a society rests, first of all, on a change in social conditions, an example being the 'reduction of labour to a minimum'.[88] Furthermore, his analysis of technology as an original means of self-preservation, discussed in Chapter 5, suggests that a better world may come about when technological progress is aimed at human progress instead of being an end in itself. And his analysis of the false needs created by the culture industry implies that a good society revolves around the satisfaction of the real needs of people (of which his above-discussed analyses of happiness and satisfaction provide us with examples), not around the commodified and standardized desires that are created by consumption culture.

Another hint is found in Adorno's analysis of the moral addendum, which was discussed in Chapter 8.[89] He argues that the guiding force behind the construction of a good society is the need to abolish suffering:

> It is not up to the individual sufferer to abolish suffering or to mitigate it to a degree which theory cannot anticipate, to which it can set no limit. This job is up solely to the species, to which the individual belongs even where he subjectively renounces it and is objectively thrust into the absolute loneliness of a helpless subject. All activities of the species point to its continued physical existence... Even the steps which society takes to exterminate itself are at the same time absurd acts of unleashed self-preservation.... Confronted with such steps, their purpose – and this alone makes a society a society – calls for it to be so organized as the productive forces would directly permit it here and now, and as the conditions of production on either side relentlessly prevent it. The *telos* of such an organization of society would be to negate the physical suffering of even the least of its members, and to negate the internal reflexive forms of that suffering. By now, this negation of the interest of all can be realized only in a solidarity that is transparent to itself and all the living.[90]

This passage contains two more characteristics of Adorno's ideas about a good society. First, he argues that constructing such a society is a communal act: only as a community of people can we change the conditions under which we live. Adorno links this idea to the drive to self-preservation: even though in modernity this drive has transformed into hostility towards otherness, it is this same drive that underlies the need to abolish suffering. We have seen in Chapter 4, after all, that Adorno links the constitution of the self to the ability to foresee danger and protect oneself against possible threats and possible suffering.

Since this drive has eventually turned into its opposite, however, Adorno is forced to argue that it has to gain a radically different shape in order to steer the course of history. He does this by connecting it to the well-being of humanity as a whole: human beings have to *collectively* organize themselves in such a way that suffering is no more. Nevertheless, this collective endeavour is still guided by the original aim of the drive to self-preservation: creating a situation in which one's existence is not defined by bare survival.

This brings us to a second aspect of Adorno's above-cited passage on the constitution of a good society: transforming one's individual drive to self-preservation into an embrace of the preservation of one's species requires a rational and self-critical moment.[91] He argues that we have to realize that the drive to self-preservation has paradoxically resulted in a corrosion of the self and that we therefore have to radically criticize this drive to stay true to its original end: the abolition of suffering. In Chapters 6 and 8 we have indeed seen that Adorno praises the critical and self-reflective aspects of Kant's philosophy.[92]

This rational insight is coupled to a different understanding of freedom. Adorno rejects the idea that every individual is separated from society or from other individuals and is therefore completely responsible for its own well-being. Instead, freedom lies in the rational realization that one is partly dependent on social and cultural processes and, therefore, on the well-being of humanity as a whole.

A last suggestion regarding the organization of a good society is found in Adorno's descriptions of metaphysical experiences. In the above-cited passage in *Minima Moralia* about animals and children, for example, he refers to children's games and argues that children unconsciously 'rehearse the right life' by overcoming second nature and siding 'with use-value rather than exchange value'.[93]

This means that metaphysical experiences offer us flashes of a different relationship between subject and object, self and world, human beings and nature. In a good society, they show us, human beings do not seek to violently dominate themselves and others, 'hitting out blindly at other people'.[94] In such a society, the subject approaches the world with openness and respect, limiting its tendency to dominate and tempering its need to control and subsume. It treats nature, the environment, the body and life as fragile and vulnerable and gives preponderance to the object, thereby piercing through the wrong veil that is projected upon the world by the culture industry.

Self-denial and society

Before we arrive at a conclusion, I want to develop a critical analysis of these ideas by arguing that they bring us back to Schopenhauer, more specifically to the latter's understanding of *self-denial*. We have seen in Chapters 5 and 6 that Adorno is quite ambivalent about the true nature of the dominating tendencies of the rational self. At places he approaches the modern subject as historical through and through and therefore as a product of historical and social circumstances. At other places, however, he infuses his Hegelian observations with materialist and naturalist claims, comparing the faculty of reason to the teeth of a bear and the feeler of a snail.

This latter observation has severe consequences for Adorno's understanding of the construction of a good society. Since he argues at several places that things have never been better; that there has never been a Golden Age or an exemplary and 'balanced' state of nature[95] ('if any harmony of subject and object should have prevailed in those days, it was a harmony like the most recent one: pressure-born and brittle'[96]); that human beings have always and everywhere dominated others and their environment, enslaved by a drive to self-preservation that in the modern age might have turned against itself and others more aggressively than ever but that has always been present in a hostile manner, he dramatically limits the possibilities of constituting a social state in which things are organized in a better way. And this suggests, in turn, that Adorno's above-discussed idea that the drive to self-preservation needs to be embedded in the preservation of one's species requires a complete change within the human self.

Like Schopenhauer, Adorno has to argue that a good society can only come about once human beings overcome that which has, until the present moment, tragically defined the course of human history: a violent drive to self-preservation and a need to dominate nature. Even though Schopenhauer does not stress the role of rationality and describes rather different roads towards salvation, his emphasis on denial and the fundamental sense in which the self has to turn against itself to better its own life returns in Adorno's ideas on the constitution of a good society. Furthermore, even though both develop rather different analyses of the exact nature of aesthetic contemplation, their ideas on aesthetics refer to similar mechanisms. We have seen that Schopenhauer argues that aesthetic contemplation provides us with one of the clearest models of a change within the human self, since the subject that contemplates art has renounced its willing nature, its need to control and dominate and to perceive everything and everyone only in relation to its own ego. Adorno's analyses of aesthetics, in which the notions of Platonic Ideas or pure will-less knowledge are absent, hints at a similar overcoming of egotism and a constitution of openness, forming the basis for the construction of a world in which violence and suffering are no more.

This Schopenhauerian aspect of Adorno's metaphysical and social observations is a result of the latter's above-mentioned attempt to do justice to two rather different approaches to the human self: on the one hand, naturalist observations on the rise of rationality as an evolutionary tool, and on the other historicist claims regarding the specific and therefore changeable nature of instrumental rationality. This uncomfortable tension is insightfully put into words by Peter Dews:

> In certain respects Adorno's conception of the ethical, in both its positive and its negative aspects, can be seen as an attempt to combine an account of autonomy (and its perversion) inherited from German Idealism with anti-rationalist and proto-naturalist influences stemming from Schopenhauer. But to achieve this fusion, he must historicize the metaphysics of the arch-pessimist. ... Adorno's framing narrative recounts the rise of instrumentality, the claim that 'in the historical form in which we encounter it to his day, reason is both reason *and* unreason in one'. Within this context, Schopenhauer's descriptions of the 'blind unstoppable drive' of the will, the futile competition of egoisms in which we are caught up, regains its evocative power.[97]

Whereas Schopenhauer, as we have seen, tries to combine naturalist and materialist observations on the world, human beings and animals with the philosophical tradition of idealism, Adorno seeks to go even further by attempting to combine not only Kant's understandings of autonomy and rational reflection with Schopenhauer's naturalism, but also to embed this combination of two contradicting lines of thinking in a historicist and critical way of thinking that follows from Hegel and Marx. Adorno therefore infuses Schopenhauer's naturalism with a psychoanalytic analysis of how our bodily experiences and needs are always entwined with social categories and with historically shaped ideas. Whereas Schopenhauer, in other words, argues that piercing through the *veil of Maya* enables us to realize that the *principium individuationis* is illusory, Adorno claims that a removal of the veil of commodification allows us to realize that we are unfree.

Nevertheless, Adorno's emphasis on the overpowering nature of several of these mechanisms makes his social thought, in places, come dangerously close to Schopenhauer's fatalism, which made Lukács place both philosophers in the Grand Hotel Abyss. Perhaps the best illustration of this uncomfortable tension within Adorno's philosophy can be found in the last paragraph of *Dialectic of Enlightenment* called 'In the Genesis of Stupidity', the same paragraph in which intelligence is compared to the feeler of a snail, as discussed in Chapter 5. Echoing Freud's observations on scar-formation, Horkheimer and Adorno there observe:

> Stupidity is a scar. It can relate to one faculty among many or to them all, practical and mental. Every partial stupidity in a human being marks a spot where the awakening play of muscles has been inhibited instead of fostered. With the inhibition, the vain repetition of unorganized, awkward attempts originally began. The child's endless questions are already a sign of a secret pain, a serious question to which it has found no answer and which it cannot frame in its proper form. The repetition half resembles playful determination, as when a dog endlessly leaps against a door it has not learned how to open, finally giving up if the handle is too high, and half corresponds to hopeless compulsion, as when a lion paces endlessly up and down in its cage or a neurotic repeats the defence reaction which has already proved futile. If the child has wearied of its repetitions, or if the thwarting has been too brutal, its attention can turn in another direction; the child is richer in experience, as one says, but at the point where its impulse has been blocked a scar can easily be left behind, a slight callus where the surface is numb. Such scars lead to deformations. They can produce 'characters,' hard and capable; they can produce stupidity, in the form of deficiency symptoms, blindness, or impotence, if they merely stagnate, or in the form of malice, spite, and fanaticism, if they turn cancerous within.... Like the genera within the series of fauna, the intellectual gradations within the human species, indeed, the blind spots within the same individual, mark the point where hope has come to a halt and in their ossification bear witness to what holds all living things in thrall.[98]

Dialectic of Enlightenment ends with these sentences, which illustrate my claim that Adorno is torn between two different ways of thinking: on the one hand he leaves open the possibility that hope can be placed in a child once it is educated and stimulated on an intellectual level, once its impulses and needs are not 'thwarted'. On the other hand he suggests that human beings almost necessarily develop 'blind spots', driven by impulsive needs that are destined not to be answered in civilization and therefore to develop into 'stupidity' – by which he refers to the formation of ideas and feelings that constitute xenophobia, racism, anti-Semitism and barbarism. These blind spots are characterized as 'scars', which implies that they become part of the body, of the materialistic dimension of one's being. Comparing the impulsiveness of a child with the behaviour of animals – again, animals return over and over in the *Dialectic of Enlightenment* to illustrate human behaviour – and arguing that the development of a 'character' is necessarily bound to the formation of these bodily scars and, thus, the repression of instincts and impulses, Adorno's negative diagnosis of modernity borders on the pessimism of Schopenhauer.

But it would be wrong to conclude that Adorno chooses to go one of these ways, which makes him different from Schopenhauer. Staying true to the method of negative dialectics and to the ideals of Critical Theory, he tries to hold open both roads, each criticizing the other. This results in a point of view that implies that change is extremely difficult, but that fatalistically embracing the idea that all hope is lost is equally one-sided. A similar idea returns in his discussion of the drive to self-preservation: on the one hand, he turns almost completely against this drive by arguing that it has always forced human beings to dominate themselves and their environment. On the other, he claims that hope lies precisely in the never-realized but nevertheless present aims of this drive: the need to abolish suffering and to increase the well-being of humanity as a whole. This same tension characterizes Adorno's analysis of technology: on the one hand, technological progress has brought us the atom bomb, chemical weapons and refined ways to monitor, control and manipulate people. On the other hand, it enables us to produce medicine, for example, or to better living conditions in poverty-stricken areas. Whereas Schopenhauer's metaphysical monism forces him to argue that human beings have to completely overcome their selves in order to find peace, Adorno's historical and dialectical critique, in other words, allows him to avoid Schopenhauer's absolutism and to claim that hope can still be found in traces of a self that has to radically change but *not* be completely denied.

It is this same negative dialectical approach that is reflected by Adorno's ambivalent stance towards Schopenhauer. Whereas he criticizes him, as we have seen, for not paying attention to the influence of history and for dogmatically denying the notions of rational critique, social change and human autonomy, he praises him, as we have seen as well, for forming a radical antipode to Kant and Hegel and confronting them with the naïve nature of their thought by emphasizing the tragic implications of naturalistic approaches to human beings, and with grim but realistic observations regarding the suffering that takes place in the world.

It is only by refusing to choose either way, Adorno suggests, that progress can be made, since progress can only be made once it is accompanied by a constant critical stance towards the status quo. And this critical stance, Critical Theory and *Negative Dialectics* teach us, can only be kept alive if we do not dogmatically embrace one idea, one interpretation, one theory, but keep open our perspectives on reality by preserving, instead of overcoming, a dialectical tension between different approaches.

Conclusion

I want to highlight a famous passage in *Negative Dialects* in conclusion:

> At its most materialistic, materialism comes to agree with theology. Its great desire would be the resurrection of the flesh, a desire utterly foreign to idealism, the realm of the absolute spirit. The perspective vanishing point of historic materialism would be its self-sublimation, the spirit's liberation from the primacy of material needs in their state of fulfilment. Only if the physical urge were quenched would the spirit be reconciled and would become that which it only promises while the spell of material conditions will not let it satisfy material needs.[99]

Adorno here develops the idea that the existence of hunger, pain and suffering, caused by the material conditions of society, prevents the subject from experiencing 'the resurrection of the flesh' and keeps pulling it down into a material reality of pain, suffering and survival. A good society, in other words, only comes about once no one unnecessarily suffers; once the body does not torment us anymore with directly or indirectly inflicted pain;[100] once there are no more beggars.

However, as long as the flesh has not been resurrected and the subject has not found peace with its body, we have to rely on brief metaphysical experiences to provide us with an idea of how things could be. Until this resurrection, in other words, bodily suffering and the experience of peace remain mute, geological stratums present in the background of our art, which has to express its dissatisfaction with the way of the world by way of a radicalization of the mechanisms that steer it. As Adorno writes in *Aesthetic Theory*: 'Subjective pleasure in the artwork would approximate a state of release from the empirical as from the totality of heteronomous. Schopenhauer may have been the first to realize this. The happiness gained from artworks is that of having suddenly escaped.'[101] Until the resurrection of the flesh, art merely provides us with a brief method of escape; until then happiness does not exist: it can only be alluded to by expressing its impossibility.

11
Conclusion

An animal showing a wound

I want to conclude this book by briefly describing several similarities between Schopenhauer and Adorno on the one hand and the South-African author J.M. Coetzee on the other. I will do this by highlighting an implicit theme of this study – animality – which allows me to summarize the strengths and weaknesses of my hitherto developed observations.

In Coetzee's collection of essayistic fiction *The Lives of Animals*, the title character Elizabeth Costello develops a moral outlook on the world that revolves around a Schopenhauerian compassion with human and animal suffering.[1] This outlook is based on that which Costello defines as 'the living flesh'.[2] This flesh allows us, in her view, to feel compassion with the suffering of human and non-human creatures, since it makes us equal as bodies capable of feeling pain. Like Schopenhauer, Costello merely describes this phenomenon instead of rationally defending it.

She refers to Kafka's short story *A Report to an Academy* to make this point. In this story the ape Red Peter narrates how he was captured by a hunting expedition in the African jungle, put in a cage and shipped to Europe. In order to survive, he mimicked human behaviour and eventually learned how to speak. The story revolves around the border between man and animal, not only addressing the violence done to the innocent ape by his captors, but also showing how Red Peter's becoming civilized was strictly driven by his drive to self-preservation in an environment consisting of threatening humans. Referring to the red scar that gave Red Peter his name, inflicted when he was shot and captured, Costello defines her descriptive morality as follows: 'I am not a philosopher of mind but an animal exhibiting, yet not exhibiting, to a gathering of scholars a wound, which I cover up under my clothes but touch on every word I speak.'[3]

In a short essayistic story added to Coetzee's *The Lives of Animals*, Peter Singer criticizes Coetzee's viewpoint as inconsistent and irrational. Coetzee, Singer argues, does not do justice to the fact that there is more to human existence than to non-human existence.[4] He also claims – in a manner similar to Korsgaard's defence of rational endorsement – that Coetzee's focus on compassion comes too close to the Humean idea that the basis of morality consists of rather random feelings, ignoring the rational capacities of human beings.[5]

Singer, I believe, misses the point of Coetzee's writings, and this reflects the vulnerability and, at the same time, the relevance of the moral outlook discussed in this book. Taking Adorno's insistence on the historically mediated nature of our (moral) observations into account, Coetzee's writings should be understood as products of and as critical reflections on the South Africa he grew up in. In novels like *Disgrace*, *Life and Times of Michael K.* and *Age of Iron*, Coetzee describes the same wrong whole that Adorno sketches, a whole that is as 'corpsed' as the universe of Beckett's *Endgame*. The protagonists of most of his novels live in a world characterized by institutionalized violence, by hatred and hostility, by corrupted political systems and ways of thinking that are infused with the ideological racism of *apartheid*. In his writings, the faculty of reason has been reduced to a mere tool, an instrument of the survival of one's self or group; if there is anything left of this faculty, it is only the tragic ability to reflect on one's own powerlessness.

Often, Coetzee's literary personae even struggle to remain a self at all – the protagonist of *Life and Times of Michael K.*, for example, slowly disintegrates into nothingness, illustrating Adorno's claim that no real living takes place in a whole that is false. Indeed, Coetzee himself described South Africa as characterized by 'deformed and stunted relations between human beings' and 'a deformed and stunted inner life'. He also stated: 'South African literature is a literature in bondage. It is a less than fully human literature. It is exactly the kind of literature you would expect people to write from prison.'[6]

A similar point can be made about Coetzee's reference to *A Report to an Academy*. As mentioned several times in Chapters 8 and 10, Adorno interprets Kafka's stories about animals as reflections of a world in which human beings are reduced to an animalistic state. By taking this state to the extreme, these stories form parodies of a wrong status quo that force us to reflect on that which makes us human and that which we share with animals, he observes. Animals hereby play both a parodying and an exemplary role.

Singer fails to realize that it is against the background of this wrong whole that Coetzee refers to the phenomenon of compassion and to the vulnerability of the flesh as a last, bleak, quivering remainder of connectedness. Like Adorno, furthermore, who approaches animal existence as exemplary both for moral behaviour ('having been a good animal') and for metaphysical experiences ('rien faire comme une bête'), Coetzee refers to the flesh and to animal life in an attempt to make us aware of a corporeal stratum that is repressed by overly rational approaches to morality.

Fallibility and hope

Pessimism

This brings me to the conclusion to this book. Peter Singer's failure to notice the conditions that shape Coetzee's conclusions about compassion and animal suffering reflects the vulnerability and fallibility of the moral outlook that, as I have sought to argue, both Schopenhauer and Adorno develop. Both authors conclude that we live in a world that is wrong and that most human beings fail to be moral. Furthermore, they claim that we ourselves are part of this wrongness as well and have constituted it with help of our faculty of reason. From their point of view, Singer's analysis of rational endorsement is in need of a meta-critical reflection on rationality itself, and thereby on the limits and the instrumental dimensions of our existence as rational creatures.

In defence of Singer, it could be argued that the world is not as horrible and wrong as Schopenhauer and Adorno claim, and that their philosophies revolve around an unbalanced emphasis on suffering, pain and barbarity and are, therefore, overly pessimistic. I think that it is very important to realize, however, that even though the kind of suffering that both describe has, for example, not taken place on a large scale during the last 65 years in the country in which I happen to live, it does take place in other countries. People are still tortured, people are still killed for the colour of their skin, their religious beliefs or their sexual orientation, and millions of children still grow up in social and cultural contexts defined by poverty, war, hatred and hunger. And too often these horrible aspects of the modern world are secretly or openly ignored by our own governments or by the governments with which they trade, by large corporations and economic organizations active or even based in our own countries. It may therefore be possible to find happiness if one belongs to a privileged social group or if one lives in a privileged country, but this happiness, as Adorno states in *Negative Dialectics*, 'is but a fragment of the entire happiness men are denied, and are denied by themselves'.[7]

It is also important to observe that the social and psychological mechanisms that Schopenhauer and Adorno analyse are present in those countries in which war and suffering have, for the time being, been eradicated. These mechanisms revolve around a hatred of anything that is different, and a closing off of oneself for the well-being of others; processes that result in xenophobia, racism, discrimination, homophobia and violence. Schopenhauer and Adorno's writings force us to realize that it is naïve to believe that these mechanisms have disappeared or cannot return.

Optimism

I have tried to show that it is against the background of observations on the overwhelming bleakness of the world, on the ways in which we are often enslaved by self-preservation, and on the easiness with which are able to hurt each other or treat the pain of others with indifference, that both Schopenhauer and Adorno highlight the only experiences that, in their common (on this point) view, preserve a sense of difference: bodily compassion and metaphysical flashes of otherness and connectedness.

Furthermore, Adorno defends a weak but crucial form of rational reflection that provides us with the capacity to deconstruct the walls we have built around ourselves and the rationalizations with which we too often justify hatred, violence and racism. I have also discussed that Adorno develops an image of a good or just society that partly follows from these metaphysical flashes of happiness and from his observations on morality. These two aspects make him different from Schopenhauer, whose metaphysical and ahistorical monism makes it impossible to claim that happiness can be found in the world itself and who eventually embraces a passivity that Adorno's socially oriented critique rejects.

Based on these observations, I want to conclude that Schopenhauer and Adorno both develop a moral outlook on the world rather than a rationally constructed moral system. This outlook finds its basis in a concern with the material vulnerability of other beings to pain and suffering, and is characterized by a fundamental physical abhorrence of violence. Furthermore, it springs from the observation that most, if not all people are to a large extent strangers to themselves, unable to constitute themselves as autonomous beings, since they are often overcome by and permeated with dimensions of their existence that they do not control. Schopenhauer's reflections on egotism – constituted by a self that perceives a world permeated with the *principium individuationis* and that is steered by a drive to self-preservation – or on evil personalities – torn apart by inner despair and suffering from endless and groundless pains – and Adorno's observations on a self 'blindly hitting out' at other people – permeated by a distorted drive to self-preservation and by pathological social images – are therefore first and foremost attempts to *understand* why people so often fail to care about other beings or actively hurt them.[8]

Like Coetzee's analysis of *A Report to an Academy*, the moral outlook both develop is too frail to be consistent or fully embedded in a rational system. But this frailness and this fallibility are the most convincing arguments for its necessity in a world that is still defined by the radical human catastrophes that made both Schopenhauer and Adorno characterize this world as wrong.

Notes

1 Introduction

1. NK: 212.
2. Kafka 2007: 16–17.
3. Kafka 2007: 18.
4. Kafka 2007: 18.
5. See for example Said 2003.
6. Butler 1998: 41. See for a discussion of Adorno's moral philosophy and writing style in connection with Kafka's *In the Penal Colony*: Lee 2005: 113–21.
7. NK: 213.
8. NK: 223.
9. NK: 227.
10. ND: 3.
11. Marx 2000: 173.
12. Müller-Doohm 2003: 684.
13. See also Zuidervaart 2007: 61.
14. Sebastian Gardner insightfully argues that Schopenhauer can be understood as the point at which two 'originally united strands of the enlightenment' – rationalist humanism and scientific naturalism – are separated and turned against each other, the latter unmasking the pseudo-religious nature of the former (Gardner 1999: 404). See also Dews 2008: 134–5.
15. Spierling 1985: 13.
16. WWR-II: 578. See also Janaway 1999c: 280.
17. Leibniz 2007: 69, 131–2, 139. 'If this is the best of all possible worlds, then what must the others be like?' (Voltaire 2006: 15).
18. WWR-II: 582–3.
19. ND: 361.
20. WWR-II: 583.
21. MM: 50. I have changed 'false' into 'wrong' in this translation, since this term, in my view, captures the multi-dimensional meaning of the German 'falsch' better. I will use the same translation of 'falsch' throughout this book.
22. ND: 366–7.
23. The phrase 'second nature' will be discussed in Chapter 5.
24. MM: 50 fn. See Hegel 1977: 11.
25. See also Gimmel 2011: 147.
26. This difference between Schopenhauer and Adorno, for example, is put into words by the latter in a passage on ignorance of death in *Negative Dialectics*. Adorno claims that this ignorance is a social product and criticizes Schopenhauer and Heidegger for arguing that it follows from the ahistorical nature of human beings (ND: 396).
27. See Vandenrath 1977: 15.

28. See Lukács 1980: 193.
29. See for example HF: 8. See also Früchtl 1991: 36–7.
30. See also Cartwright 1989: 55, Vandenabeele 2012: 1.
31. See Magee 1983: 350–417, Janaway 1997: 101, Maas 2010: 774–7, Vandenabeele 2012: 7, Houellebecq 2004.
32. See Rowles 2014.
33. Schopenhauer 2000e. Hannah describes this 'revolting misogynist diatribe' as 'entirely unworthy of Schopenhauer' (Hannan 2009: x). It could be argued, however, that it is precisely the ahistorical character of Schopenhauer's metaphysical essentialism as a whole that makes it possible for him to develop a totalizing analysis of the unchangeable nature of 'women in general'.
34. BM: 80.
35. WWR-II: 303.
36. For example, Schopenhauer is not mentioned in otherwise excellent studies that (partly) focus on Adorno's concern with embodiment like Lee 2005, Bernstein 2001, Zuidervaart 2007. Cook mentions Schopenhauer only once, regarding Adorno's concern with the suffering of animals (Cook 2011: 127). In *Adorno's Practical Philosophy: Living Less Wrongly* – in my view the best study of Adorno's moral philosophy available – Freyenhagen discusses Schopenhauer only briefly regarding Adorno's references to compassion (Freyenhagen 2013: 130–2). In Peter Dews' *The Idea of Evil* (2008) we do find several references to the similarities between Schopenhauer and Adorno. I mention these references throughout this book. In several studies published in German, furthermore, the similarities between the two authors are explored extensively. See Gimmel 2011, Wischke 1994, 1996, Früchtl 1991.
37. See Janaway 1999a: I. The quote is taken from MM: 153.
38. Vandenabeele 2012: 1.
39. LND: 104. Adorno criticizes Hegel and Marx for claiming that a certain amount of suffering may have been necessary for human and social development. See also Freyenhagen 2013: 69.
40. Adorno's *Doktorvater* at the University of Frankfurt, the neo-Kantian philosopher Hans Cornelius, was influenced by Schopenhauer as well. *The World as Will and Representation* actually contributed to his decision to turn away from studying the natural sciences and focus on philosophy (Müller-Doohm 2003: 108–9).
41. Jay 1973: 44.
42. Jay 1973: 44.
43. Jay 1973: 25.
44. Veauthier 1988: 593.
45. Horkheimer 1961: 19. See also Veauthier 1988: 593.
46. Horkheimer 1961: 16, 23. Peter Dews in fact notices in *The Idea of Evil* that '[t]he famous Marxist accusation that Hegel turns the world upside down, deriving reality from the Idea, occurs in numerous forms throughout [Schopenhauer's] work' (Dews 2008: 123). See also Janaway 1999c: 2–3; Vandenrath 1977.
47. See also Veauthier 1988: 594.
48. Horkheimer 1961: 19. See also Jay 1973: 105.
49. Horkheimer 1961: 13.
50. Horkheimer 1961: 14–15.

51. Horkheimer 1961:19, 21. Horkheimer 1955: 53, Horkheimer 1974b: 72–3, Veauthier 1988: 593, 598, Müller-Doohm 2003: 120.
52. Veauthier 1988: 597.
53. Horkheimer 1961: 14. Horkheimer 1955: 55, Horkheimer 1974b: 66.
54. See also Veauthier 1988: 598, Vandenrath 1977: 28.
55. Lukács 1988: 22.
56. Adorno 1991: 225–6.
57. MM: 154.
58. Büttner 2002: 115. See also Nixon 2011: 53–6, 170. Beckett's pessimistic reading of Proust was highly influenced by Schopenhauer as well (see Nixon 2011: 102; Dowd 2009: 90).
59. See Robertson 2002: 102, 117, Robertson 2004: 121–2. It has even been argued that the name of the protagonist of Kafka's *The Metamorphosis* – 'Samsa' – was inspired by Schopenhauer's references to 'Samsara', which he took from the *Upanishads* and refers to our enslavement to both our bodies and the world (see Ryan 1999). Furthermore, it has been suggested that the castle in Kafka's novel *The Castle* refers to Schopenhauer's references to the inaccessible nature of the in-itself (Zilcosky 2007). Schopenhauer writes in this context: 'We are like a man who goes round a castle, looking in vain for an entrance, and sometimes sketching the façades' (WWR-I: 99).
60. Jordan 2001: 101–2.
61. Adorno makes a similar point about Kafka, claiming that 'pessimism' and 'optimism' do not apply to his works: 'The light source that shows the world's crevices is the optimal one' (NK: 236). Even though Adorno appears to be wary of the term 'pessimism', I believe his constant focus on the horrors of the world and his emphasis on the dark and almost hopeless nature of existence make it rather difficult not to approach his writings as pessimistic in nature.
62. NK: 236.
63. Marx 1990: 103.
64. PMP: 15. See also Freyenhagen 2013: 10.
65. The phrase 'method of escape' is developed by Julian Young in a study of Schopenhauer (Young 1987: 146).
66. See WWR-I: xii.
67. See for a characterization of his own methodology and style: Adorno 1984, MM: 126–7. An interesting analysis of Adorno's style – and its similarities with Nietzsche's writings – is developed in Rose 1978. See for an emphasis on Adorno's use of exaggeration Van den Brink 1997.
68. See also Wicks 2012, Dews 2008: 124–5.
69. 'Micrology is the place where metaphysics finds a haven from totality' (ND: 407).

2 A Paradox of Transcendence and Immanence

Parts of Chapters 2 and 3 were published as a paper on Schopenhauer and Merleau-Ponty (see Peters 2013a).

1. Atwell 1995: 81. In a footnote, Atwell adds that the two French existential phenomenologists Jean-Paul Sartre and Maurice Merleau-Ponty can both be characterized as 'philosophers of the body' as well. Similar claims about

Schopenhauer can be found in two essays on his analysis of embodiment: Dörpinghaus 2000: 16, Dörflinger 2002: 43.

2. WWR-I: 3.
3. In his introduction to the first volume of *The World as Will and Representation*, Schopenhauer claims that without acquaintance with the *Fourfold Root* it is 'quite impossible' to understand his chief work 'properly' (WWR-I: xiv).
4. FR: 185.
5. See FR: 31.
6. FR: 83.
7. FR: 32.
8. FR: 32.
9. FR: 32.
10. White 1999: 67.
11. FR: 37.
12. FR: 61.
13. FR: 61.
14. BM: 211.
15. FR: 58.
16. FR: 37.
17. White argues that we could ask, especially in light of recent observations in the fields of (quantum) physics, if Schopenhauer's claim is correct that all changes in objects are *caused*: 'there are good grounds for holding that atoms can decay without cause, that matter came into existence some fifteen billion years ago, and that all causal series, like time and space themselves, had a beginning' (White 1999: 86). I do not believe this to be a very strong observation, since Schopenhauer's observations precisely make it possible to claim that the world that the subject perceives (consisting of spatiotemporal objects) is different from the way the world is 'external' to our perception of it (according to the theory White refers to, as consisting of quanta). In fact, Erwin Schrödinger, one of the fathers of quantum physics, was deeply influenced by Schopenhauer. In *Mind and Matter*, Schrödinger states, repeating the first sentence of Schopenhauer's chief work: 'The world extended in space and time is but our representation (*Vorstellung*). Experience does not give us the slightest clue of its being anything besides that, as Berkeley was well aware' (Schrödinger 2001: 135–6). Albert Einstein was also deeply influenced by Schopenhauer and based his ideas about morality on Schopenhauer's ideas on compassion (see Einstein 1997).
18. WWR-I: 104. See also Janaway 1999b: 140–71.
19. See WWR-I: 104.
20. WWR-II: 8. See also Janaway 1999b: 167. Schopenhauer hereby comes close to what Kant in *Critique of Pure Reason* describes as 'empirical idealism'. Kant attributes this idea to Berkeley and defines it as follows: 'while admitting the reality of space, [empirical idealism] denies, or at least doubts, the existence of bodies extended in it, and thus leaves us without a sufficient criterion of reality and illusion.' (Kant 2003: 278). Indeed, on the one hand Schopenhauer's strategy brings him closer to empiricism, since it analyses our direct perception of the world and ignores Kant's rationalism. On the other hand, it moves him further away from this doctrine because it cannot transcendentally guarantee the conditions of its possibility. See for an analysis of Kant and Berkeley: Janaway 1999c: 151.

21. WWR-I: 4, WWR-I: 419.
22. Kant 1977: 4.
23. Kant 1977: 51–2.
24. WWR-I: 430.
25. WWR-I: 430. Schopenhauer in fact misinterprets Kant's understanding of a 'judgment' as being, in his view, the result of an unnecessary conceptual addition to a world we *already* directly perceive. He does not realize that, for Kant, judgements are not *added* to perception but constitute perception *itself*. See also Guyer 1999: 117–18.
26. WWR-I: 25.
27. See Janaway 1999c: 170.
28. FR: 65. Schopenhauer uses the metaphor of digestion to refer to intelligence or perception several times. This metaphor found its way to Nietzsche, who understands the body, as Blondel argues in his famous work on Nietzsche, as 'a series of instincts (Instinkte) or drives (Triebe) that constitute reality as they interpret it' (Blondel 1991: 206).
29. See for example FR: 68.
30. See for example FR: 80. Schopenhauer even argues that the distinction between phenomena and things-in-themselves is based on Kant's 'discovery' that 'brain-functions' play an important role in constructing the world we perceive. He admits, however, that Kant did not make this discovery 'under this name' (WWR-I: 418).
31. WWR-II: 46–7.
32. Schopenhauer died one year before Darwin's *On the Origin of Species* was published. Although one can find ideas in Schopenhauer's works that anticipate Darwin's understanding of the origin of species – later in his life, Schopenhauer did believe that species developed out of each other – it is important to notice that his theory on species as 'fixed' and unchangeable did prohibit him from accepting the Darwinist idea that species develop gradually and through *subtle* and often almost unnoticeable changes. See also Janaway 1999c: 254–5.
33. WN 299. As an example, Schopenhauer mentions that his dog is able to 'understand' the causal relation between the pulling of a string and the moving of curtains attached to this string (FR: 89).
34. WWR-I 30. See also Wicks 2012: 156–9.
35. Spierling 1985: 32. ['The world is in my head, and my head is in the world.' – My translation.]
36. WWR-I: 3.
37. WWR-I: 19.
38. WWR-I: 20.
39. WWR-I: 20.
40. WWR-I: 30.
41. Young 1987: 3.
42. Young 1987: 12.
43. See also: Janaway 1999b: 285–6.
44. Janaway 1999c: 181.
45. Janaway 1999c: 186–7.
46. WWR-I: 30.
47. AE: 144–5.
48. AE: 145n.

49. AE: 142.
50. AE: 144n.
51. WWR-I: 19.
52. WWR-II: 13.
53. Even though Schopenhauer argues that he agrees with Kant's claims concerning the unity of apperception, he also departs from Kant by arguing that this unity is constituted by an underlying 'will' and that animals perceive this world essentially in the same unified manner. See for example WWR-II: 139.
54. SO: 249.
55. DE: 155. See also ; Müller-Doohm 2003: 157.
56. Merleau-Ponty 1958: 353. See for an analysis of Schopenhauer and Merleau-Ponty: Schmicking 2012.
57. Merleau-Ponty 1958: xxi.
58. The paradox that Schopenhauer's epistemology contains plays an important role in the idea of a 'return to the lived body' developed by French existentialist phenomenologists. In Sartre's *Being and Nothingness,* for example, it is discussed at great length (Sartre 1984: 415). Nietzsche discusses this paradox as well, even making fun of it in *Beyond Good and Evil* (See Wicks 2012: 158).
59. Merleau-Ponty, for example, argues that 'space' is not an *a priori* category, but can only be understood once we take our bodily existence into account (Merleau-Ponty 2004: 42).
60. Merleau-Ponty 1964: 16.
61. Merleau-Ponty 1964: 16.
62. AE: 157.

3 The World-as-Will

1. WWR-II: 584.
2. Schopenhauer 2000d: 309.
3. Schmied 1996: 70.
4. Deleuze 2005: 17.
5. As quoted in Deleuze 2005: 17. See also Schmied 1996: 72.
6. In Chapter 9 I discuss the idea of a development of several 'stages' within Schopenhauer's philosophy, also paying attention to the observation that his discussion of the world-as-representation forms a stepping-stone towards a discussion of the world-as-will.
7. Simmel 1991: 20.
8. FR: 1.
9. WWR-I: 417–8.
10. WWR-I: 419.
11. From a certain perspective, Schopenhauer's dualism between different ways of approaching the body – as a scientific and individual object, and as a living, breathing and developing entity – is similar to the dualism described within the existentialist phenomenological tradition. However, Schopenhauer's metaphysics eventually makes his notion of Will different from the 'lived

body' as described by existential phenomenologists like Merleau-Ponty. See for a conceptualization of these two understandings of the body: Leder 1998.

12. WWR-I: 419.
13. WWR-I: 5.
14. WWR-I: 105.
15. WWR-I: 99.
16. WWR-I: 103.
17. WWR-I: 112.
18. WWR-II: 248. In *Phenomenology of Perception*, Merleau-Ponty makes the same observation regarding this 'relation': 'the relationships between my decision and my body are, in movement, magic ones' (Merleau-Ponty 1958: 108). In his *Philosophical Investigations*, furthermore, Wittgenstein discusses the difference between 'doing' and 'willing' by referring to the act of raising one's arm (Wittgenstein 1958: §612–27).
19. See also Simmel 1991: 23. In Chapter 3, I will return to this aspect of Schopenhauer's discussion of Will, which follows from his observation that Kant is not able to make sense of what it means to act freely, since acting freely means that one has to bridge the gap between the intelligible and the practical realms.
20. WWR-II: 298.
21. WWR-II: 513.
22. WWR-II: 514.
23. See also Janaway 1997: 38.
24. See also Nussbaum 1999: 347.
25. FR: 185.
26. WWR-I: 104–5.
27. WWR-I: 162. Schopenhauer uses the terms 'microcosm' and 'macrocosm' as well in his essay on morality (BM: 133).
28. WWR-I: 332.
29. WWR-II: 325–6.
30. Spierling 1985: 35. ['This leap from psychological willing to thing-in-itself, from an empirical to a metaphysical point of view' – My translation.]
31. See for example Janaway 1997: 33, 107.
32. Lukács 1980: 189. See also Young 1987: 63.
33. Lukács 1980: 188.
34. ND: 403.
35. See for an insightful discussion of Nietzsche's critique: Young 2009: 162.
36. An important discussion of this idea is found in Foucault's *History of Sexuality* (see Foucault 1990; 1998a; 1998b1990b). See also: Butler 1998.
37. See Magee 1983: 144.
38. WWR-I: 108.
39. WWR-II: 318. See also Young 1987: 65. A similar point of critique could be formulated against Hannan who, in support of Schopenhauer, argues that 'even today chemists find it difficult to avoid attributing a certain "personality" to every element' (Hannan 2009: 24). Using the analogy of personal behaviour to describe chemical reactions, of course, is fundamentally different from claiming that these elements consist of a metaphysical force,

let alone claiming that this force is not fundamentally different from the desires we experience as human beings.

40. Simmel 1991: 24.
41. Simmel 1991: 24.
42. Simmel 1991: 25.
43. Simmel 1991: 33.
44. WWR-II: 196.
45. WWR-II: 196.
46. MS: 64. ['Being in itself in human beings.' – My translation.]
47. Young also points out that Schopenhauer first affirms and then denies a direct access to the *an sich* (Young 1987: 33).
48. WWR-II: 197.
49. BM: 206.
50. WWR-I: 108.
51. Young 1987: 31.
52. Young 1987: 31–2.
53. Simmel 1991: 25.
54. MS: 36. ['However, this is thing-in-itself in just a relative sense, meaning in comparison with appearance: – and this, in turn, is appearance only in its relation to thing-in-itself. It is also a brain-phenomenon. I have never said, however, what the thing-in-itself stands outside of any relation, because I do not know this.' – My translation.]
55. WN: 373.
56. In this book, I will follow Payne's translation and use the word 'compassion', even though this term, in my view, does not completely capture what Schopenhauer means. Gerard Mannion's study *Schopenhauer, Religion and Morality: the Humble Path to Ethics* contains an interesting discussion of the different translations of *Mitleid* into either 'pity', 'sympathy', 'compassion' or 'empathy'. Mannion argues that 'compassion' is an accurate translation of *Mitleid*, since 'compassion' does not imply the superiority inherent to the notion of 'pity' – in Chapter 6, I return to this issue in relation to Adorno's critical analysis of compassion. The concept of 'sympathy', in turn, does not include the 'suffering' (*leiden*) that we feel 'with' or 'in' the other that is implied by the notion of *Mitleid*. Mannion also argues that 'empathy' implies that one participates in the suffering other in an imaginative sense (Mannion 2003: 209). These claims are not undisputed, however. Adam Smith, for example, famously defines the process underlying sympathy in *The Theory of Moral Sentiments* as follows: 'What at first disturbs us is not the object of the senses, but the idea of the imagination. [...I]t is an idea, therefore, which occasions our uneasiness' (Smith 2007: 36). Passions originating in the body, in Smith's view, 'excite either no sympathy at all, or such a degree of it, as is altogether disproportioned to the violence of what is felt by the sufferer' (Smith 2007: 35). In contrast with Mannion's ideas, we could therefore also think of the concept of 'empathy', which bears a naturalistic and biological aura that makes it different from concepts like 'sympathy' or 'compassion'. Dutch biologist Frans de Waal, for example, states in *The Age of Empathy*: 'Empathy is an automated response over which we have limited control' (De Waal 2009: 43).
57. WWR-II: 602.

58. WWR-II: 602.
59. BM: 166.
60. BM: 166.
61. BM: 147. See also Came 2012: 244.
62. See BM: 205.
63. BM: 209.
64. See BM: 209.
65. BM: 166.
66. BM: 211.
67. See WWR-I: 373.
68. In his introduction to Schopenhauer's lectures on morality, Volker Spierling develops an interesting metaphor to illustrate this aspect of Schopenhauer's metaphysics. He presents the world-as-will as the body of an 'Unendlichfüßler' or 'infinipede', each foot being a living creature. As bodies, these creatures are connected and therefore able experience compassion with each other. See Spierling 1985: 28–9.
69. This is a central idea of Horkheimer's understanding of materialism. See for example Horkheimer's discussion of the position of needs and suffering within the doctrine of materialism in Horkheimer 1972: 44. See also: Schmidt 2004:144n.
70. Lukács 1980: 188.
71. For this reason, Cartwright even argues that Schopenhauer's metaphysical and 'magical' explanation of compassion should be replaced with a psychological and scientific one (Cartwright 2009: 150). I do not agree, however. Cartwright too easily assumes that Schopenhauer would sacrifice the metaphysical nature of Will and of the phenomenon of compassion to psychological and scientific observations. This would not do justice to the specific nature of Schopenhauer's understanding of compassion, or to the fundamental role that it plays within his philosophy as a whole. See also Mannion 2003: 207.
72. Cartwright 2009: 143.
73. See for example WWR-II: 600.
74. See also Janaway 199b: 282–3.
75. Many examples of compassion occurring between human and non-human animals can be found in the works of Frans de Waal. For example, De Waal mentions experiments with rhesus monkeys who 'literally starve themselves to death to avoid inflicting pain on others' (De Waal 2006: 29).
76. BM: 175.
77. BM: 176.
78. WWR-I: 107.

4 Irrationalism and Pessimism

1. Mishima 2003: 22.
2. WWR-I: 311.
3. As quoted in Stokes 1975: 184.
4. Mishima 2003: 38.
5. Mishima 2003: 11.

6. As quoted in Young 1988: 85.
7. Lukács 1980:191.
8. Young 1988: 86.
9. Young 1988: 86.
10. Young 1988: 86. See also Janaway 1999c: 274–5.
11. Young 1988: 87.
12. WWR-II: 583.
13. WWR-I: 312.
14. WWR-II: 580.
15. WWR-II: 507.
16. WWR-II: 586. In Chapter 8 we will see that Samuel Beckett often refers to this line as well. In light of statements like these, Bryan Magee's claim that Schopenhauer's philosophy does not necessarily entail pessimism is not very convincing. Magee argues that pessimism is a rather subjective perspective on a reality that is in itself neither good nor bad, which means that a philosopher who analyses this reality cannot defend optimism or pessimism (Magee 1983: 13).
17. WWR-II: 573.
18. WWR-II: 634.
19. See also Young 1987: 137 and further.
20. WWR-II: 575.
21. See 1999b: 325, 328.
22. WWR-II: 586.
23. DS: 291.
24. DS: 297.
25. Simmel 1991: 22.
26. DS: 292.
27. Young 1988: 87.
28. Young 1988: 89–90.
29. WWR-I: 404.
30. See also Foucault 1994.
31. WWR-II: 548.
32. See WWR-II: 548.
33. See WWR-II: 540–50.
34. WWR-II: 546.
35. WWR-II: 533.
36. WWR-I: 364. Peter Dews rightly points out that Schopenhauer here anticipates the insights of psychoanalysis: 'Psychoanalysts, even from widely differing traditions, have concurred that evil is best understood as the attempt to inflict one's own experience of evacuation of meaning on others' (Dews 2008: 133).
37. Young 1988: 89–90.
38. Korsgaard 2009: xi.
39. Korsgaard 2006: 112.
40. Korsgaard 2009: 118.
41. Korsgaard 1996: 91.
42. Korsgaard 1996: 94.
43. Kant 2004: 99.
44. Kant 2004: 102.

45. Kant 2003: 304
46. Kant 2003: 304.
47. Kant 2003: 252.
48. WWR-I: 507
49. FW: 49.
50. FW: 98–9
51. WN: 95.
52. WN: 32.
53. WN: 34.
54. WN: 37.
55. WWR-II: 298.
56. Atwell 1990: 35.
57. FW: 33.
58. WN: 18.
59. WWRI: 300.
60. Freud claimed that Schopenhauer's notion of 'Will' was 'equivalent to the mental instincts of psychoanalysis' (as quoted in Zaretsky 2005: 130). Gardner convincingly argues, however, that we should not too easily equate Schopenhauer's 'Will' with Freud's 'unconscious'. Whereas the former refers to a wide range of experiences, instincts and forces, the latter consists of motivational states. And whereas the former transcends the individual being, the latter does not (see Gardner 1999: 380–3). See also Atzert 2012.
61. WWR-II: 135.
62. WWR-II: 136.
63. WN: 94.
64. WWR-II: 369.
65. WWR-II: 259.
66. WWR-II: 213.
67. See for example Atwell 1990: 57; Janaway 1999c: 243; Janaway 1999b: 339.
68. Young 1988: 95.
69. Young 1988: 91.
70. Young 1988: 96.
71. WN: 97.
72. WN: 99.
73. See also Janaway 1999c: 245.
74. BM: 83.
75. BM: 131.
76. BM: 131.
77. BM: 132.
78. BM: 132.
79. WWR-II: 577. See Hobbes 1983: 24.
80. DS: 300.
81. Lukács 1980: 193. A similar point can be made about Schopenhauer's infamous essay 'On Women' (Schopenhauer 2000e). The essentialist nature of Schopenhauer's observations on biology, sexuality and the human character makes it possible for him to develop a totalizingly negative analysis of 'women in general'. Following Lukács, this essentialist representation can be understood as a metaphysical affirmation and a philosophical apologetic of social discourses and conditions that constitute sexism and misogyny.

82. WWR-I: 347–8.
83. WWR-I: 345.
84. WWR-I: 349.
85. I therefore disagree with Bishop, who argues that Schopenhauer's discussion of the world-as-representation contains social critique: 'close attention to the text reveals there are also indications that, by the "world", Schopenhauer intends to include, and perhaps concentrate on, the social sphere – as we might call it, "the way of the world". After all, Schopenhauer underscores that he is talking about the world as it appears; and so, on one level, his great philosophical treatise is also a commentary on social mores and social interaction' (Bishop 2003: 416). Bishop does not take the naturalistic and ahistorical nature of Schopenhauer's philosophy into account: even animals, Schopenhauer argues, perceive the world-as-representation. It therefore goes too far to argue that the world-as-representation consists of 'social mores'. See for an insightful discussion of Schopenhauer's political ideas: Jordan 2009.
86. WWR-I: 350.
87. WWR-I: 350.
88. Several aspects of Schopenhauer's own life point in the same direction. Famously, he lent his opera glasses to a Prussian officer during the popular uprising in 1848, giving the officer a better view of those he tried to shoot. Furthermore, Schopenhauer's testament contained the wish to give a part of his money to an organization that assisted soldiers who fought in 1848. Schopenhauer's political ideas, these biographical events confirm, follow most of all from a distrust of human beings, a cynical rejection of the ideal of social change and an emphasis on state control to keep irrational and hostile individuals at bay.
89. Horkheimer 1955: 55; 1961: 14; 1974: 66.
90. See also Janaway 1999c: 13.
91. As quoted in Dews 2008: 124.
92. Horkheimer 1974b: 81.
93. Janaway 1999c: 286.
94. See also Dews 2008: 124–5. This conclusion ties in with recent discoveries made in the fields of biology and neurology. See for explorations of this idea: Damasio 2005; Swaab 2014.
95. Sebastian Gardner argues how Schopenhauer's philosophy is 'the primary point at which enlightenment rationalism registers the impact of naturalism' (Gardner 1999: 404).

5 The Whole Is the Wrong

Parts of Chapters 5, 6 and 8 were published as a paper on Adorno's moral philosophy (see Peters 2013b).

1. Beckett 2009: 20.
2. M: 117.
3. UE: 273.
4. HF: 113
5. See also Cook 2011: 91.
6. LND: 122.
7. Améry 1980:12.

8. LND: 120.
9. Habermas 1990: 106.
10. ND: 321.
11. DE: 36–7.
12. ND: 320.
13. ND: 355.
14. DE: 46–7.
15. DE: 184.
16. DE: 213.
17. WN: 263.
18. DE: 53.
19. DE: 43.
20. DE: 71.
21. Freud 1961: 84.
22. DE: 192.
23. DE: 193.
24. ND: 389.
25. Whitebook 2004: 62.
26. HF: 13.
27. Horkheimer 1974a: 119.
28. HF: 13.
29. HF: 169.
30. See Marx 1990 163–77.
31. Marx 1990: 164–5.
32. Marx 1990: 164.
33. Marx 1990: 165.
34. Marx 1990: 168.
35. Marx 1990: 169.
36. Marx 1990: 165.
37. Marx 1990: 168.
38. Lukács 1968: 128.
39. Lukács 1968: 129.
40. ND: 262.
41. PMP: 176.
42. In Jay Bernstein's famous work on Adorno's ethics we find perhaps the most comprehensive discussion of this kind of thinking (Bernstein 2001). See also Freyenhagen 2013: 41–51.
43. ND: 183.
44. See for example Adorno 2009: 26. See for an analysis of Heidegger's ideas on embodiment Levin 1999. A similar critique could be formulated against Merleau-Ponty's analysis of 'the flesh' in his posthumously published *The Visible and the Invisible* (Merleau-Ponty 1968).
45. Adorno 1993: 148.
46. EA: 29.
47. M: 116; ND: 320.
48. HF: 15.
49. DE: 119.

50. Adorno 1998b: 76.
51. This observation, of course, returns in several forms in feminist discourse. See for an insightful discussion of the rather uncomfortable relation between Adorno's (in places) quite essentialist thoughts on gender and femininity on the one hand, and several feminist theories on the other: Lee 2005: 123–50.
52. Adorno 1998b: 72.
53. Adorno 1998b: 73. Adorno herewith implicitly criticizes Herbert Marcuse's ideas on sexual liberation (see Marcuse 1974).
54. Adorno 1998b: 73.
55. Adorno 1998b: 77. In 'The Schema of Mass Culture' Adorno furthermore describes how the modern experience of the body is to a high extent influenced and permeated by the culture industry, even referring to the body as a 'slave': 'In the freedom which he exercises over his body the individual confirms what he is inflicting upon this slave the same injustice he has already endured at the violent hands of society' (Adorno 2001b: 89).
56. ND: 362.
57. Marx 1990: 165.
58. MM: 15.
59. Nietzsche 1974.
60. MM: 15.
61. Müller-Doohm 2003: 518. Adorno values the idea that authors like Nietzsche, Schopenhauer and Kierkegaard wrote before philosophy became academically organized and were therefore able to freely focus on matters concerning life and existence (Müller-Doohm 2003: 187–8). A similar focus returns in the unacademic and almost playful methodology and focus of *Minima Moralia*.
62. ND: 363.
63. EA: 30.
64. MM: 26.
65. ND: 219.
66. ND: 297.
67. BM: 132.
68. ND: 219.
69. See HF: 235
70. MM: 153–4.
71. MM: 154. In *On the Will in Nature*, for example, Schopenhauer observes that consciousness is clear when directed at the world-as-representation, but confronted with darkness once directed inwardly: 'on the *outside*; great clarity and illumination spread themselves before the gaze of the consciousness. But on the inside it is dark like a thoroughly blackened telescope. No a priori proposition illuminates the night of its interior; these lighthouses shine only toward the outside' (WN: 22–3).
72. UE: 267.
73. MM: 50. Translation amended. One of the few authors describing this similarity between Schopenhauer and Adorno is Peter Dews, who convincingly argues that Adorno's claim that 'the subjectivity of human beings is determined by society' can be understood as a socio-historical version of Schopenhauer's metaphysical monism (Dews 2008: 201).

6 The Twitching of the Hand

1. M: 144.
2. LND: 122.
3. HF: 121.
4. Habermas 1990: 129.
5. See for a discussion of this critique Benhabib 1986: 168; Hammer 2006: 113.
6. HF: 8.
7. DE: xvi.
8. DE: xvi.
9. PMP: 151.
10. Kant 1990: 17.
11. In an interview entitled 'Erziehung zur Mündigkeit', Adorno discusses this historical and social approach to the question 'What is enlightenment?' at length (Adorno 1971: 144).
12. ND: 31.
13. EA: 21.
14. ND: 365.
15. PMP: 103.
16. HF: 158.
17. ND: 41.
18. EA: 23.
19. PMP: 108.
20. SO: 254–5.
21. PMP: 133.
22. ND: 231.
23. ND: 227.
24. ND: 228.
25. ND: 228.
26. See for a careful analysis of Adorno's reading of Kant and a defence of Kant's understanding of freedom: Jütten 2012.
27. ND: 230.
28. ND: 389.
29. ND: 229.
30. ND: 203.
31. Hammer 2006: 117.
32. AE: 155.
33. HF: 231–5. See also Hammer 2006: 118.
34. ND: 230.
35. ND: 228.
36. ND: 228–9.
37. HF: 235.
38. See also Cook 2012: 54; Lee 2005: 7; Hammer 2006: 118–19.
39. ND: 228.
40. Whitebook 2004: 62.
41. Whitebook 2004: 73.
42. ND: 219.
43. ND: 219.
44. See also ND: 219.

7 *Neminem Laede* – Injure No One

1. DE: 76.
2. Sade 1965: 137–8.
3. BM: 55.
4. BM: 63.
5. See BM: 85–7.
6. See for example Mannion 2003: 123.
7. PMP: 151.
8. See Mannion 2003: 132.
9. PMP: 133.
10. See also Cartwright 1989: 54.
11. WN: 373.
12. BM: 1.
13. WWR-I: 271.
14. BM: 130.
15. BM: 75.
16. BM: 150.
17. Schopenhauer 1987: 263. See also Cartwright 1989: 56; Spierling 1985: 13; Ray Singh 2007: 112–13.
18. Schopenhauer 200b: 212.
19. BM: 144.
20. DS: 297.
21. WWR-I: 325.
22. Spierling 1985: 16. ['Schopenhauer "blocks" philosophy by positioning corporeal pain in its way.' – My translation.]
23. Hume 2003: 295. There are many parallels between Schopenhauer's moral philosophy and the theories developed by authors belonging to the tradition of Scottish enlightenment. Francis Hutcheson, for example, claims in a rather Schopenhauerian fashion that 'ought' is an 'unlucky word in morals' (Hutcheson 2002: XX).
24. Hume 1983: 87.
25. Korsgaard 1996: 146.
26. Korsgaard 1996: 153–4.
27. WWR-I: 393. Examples of the beneficial and creative aspects of suffering and pain can be found in many artistic works. A good example is Oscar Wilde's *De Profundis*, the epistle he wrote when imprisoned in 1897. The idea that suffering contains 'truth' because of its direct and inescapable reality plays an important role in this work (Wilde 1954: 161). A similar idea was developed by Yukio Mishima (Mishima 2003: 38).
28. See for a similar analysis in the context of Adorno's moral philosophy: Bernstein 2001: 406.
29. BM: 176.
30. Korsgaard 1996: 150.
31. Korsgaard 1996: 152.
32. Korsgaard 1996: 154.
33. Recent studies show that compassion is not an uncommon phenomenon in non-human animals. See De Waal 2009.
34. Korsgaard 2008: 205.

35. Kant 2011: 25.
36. Korsgaard 2008: 204.
37. Korsgaard 1996: 154.
38. See for an interesting exploration of this idea Maurice Hamington's *Embodied Care: Jane Addams, Maurice Merleau-Ponty, and Feminist Ethics*. Hamington focuses on the ethical notion of 'care', which follows, in his view, from Merleau-Ponty's observations on embodied perception and intercorporeity (Hamington 2004). See also Mazis 2006.
39. See BM: 143.
40. BM: 144.
41. See for example BM: 69, 149.
42. BM: 150–1.
43. See BM: 150.
44. BM: 187.
45. FW: 55.
46. BM: 132.
47. WWR-I: 397–80.
48. DE: 80.
49. DE: 80.
50. PMP: 173. See also Freyenhagen 2013: 58, 130–2; Früchtl 1991: 38.
51. DE: 80.
52. DE: 81. In *The Authoritarian Personality* Adorno analyses a person whose feelings of pity towards others, in this case African Americans, are entwined with a tendency to humiliate (Adorno 1955: 699–700). Freyenhagen discusses the example of humanitarian aid in this context, see Freyenhagen 2013: 58, 131. It could be argued that the development of this kind of aid is often used as a marketing tool to better the image of individuals or companies. Furthermore, it might function as an excuse that overshadows the fact that structural changes (on a political, economic and social level) are needed to eradicate the suffering that takes place in the world.
53. DE: 81.
54. A similar critique of *Mitleid* as masked egotism was formulated by Ludwig Feuerbach (see Früchtl 1991: 39).
55. DE : 79–80.
56. Nietzsche 1974: 88.
57. Nietzsche 1997: 133.
58. PMP: 173.
59. Nietzsche 1968: 130.
60. See, for a well-argued defence of Schopenhauer against Nietzsche, Mannion 2003: 206.
61. See also Cornell 1987; Früchtl 1991; Freyenhagen 2013: 132n.
62. See Nietzsche 1968: 130.
63. See Scheler 1979: 52, 54.
64. Scheler 1979: 53.
65. See also Cartwright 1981: 144, 147; Mannion 2003: 203.
66. See WWR-II: 575.

8 Being a Good Animal

1. Oppenhheimer 2012.
2. Oppenhheimer 2012.
3. Oppenhheimer 2012.
4. Jay Bernstein quotes a horrifying 1943 address to the SS by Heinrich Himmler, which contains similar arguments to rationalize one's feelings of doubt away. Himmler argues that the 'task' of the German people (the extermination of the Jews) is 'terrible' and that 'ordinary human compassion' would prevent it (Bernstein 2001: 409). By rationally suppressing compassion for suffering others, by rationally putting the drive for self-preservation on a pedestal as one with the preservation of one's *Volk* and one's *Reich*; by deliberately making oneself into an entwinement of nature and rationality, Himmler claimed that the soldiers of the SS could prepare themselves for the Final Solution.
5. Oppenhheimer 2012.
6. MM: 19.
7. MM: 39.
8. UE: 275. Translation amended.
9. Adorno 2003a: 162. See for a discussion of different interpretations of this often misinterpreted claim Clendinnen 2002: 166.
10. PMP: 166.
11. PMP: 165.
12. Bernstein 2001: 1.
13. DE: 90.
14. See also Schweppenhäuser 2004: 328.
15. PMP: 82.
16. PMP: 104
17. PMP: 105.
18. See for a brief but clear discussion of these two arguments against Kant: Freyenhagen 2008: 105.
19. PMP: 158.
20. DE: 69.
21. PMP: 108.
22. PMP: 97.
23. PMP: 120.
24. See Hammer 2006: 117.
25. See for a discussion of Adorno's reading of Kant: Hearfield 2004; and for a thorough and strong critique of Adorno's Kant-critique: Freyenhagen 2006: 432–3; Freyenhagen 2013: 102–20.
26. See also Bernstein 2001: 413.
27. PMP: 165.
28. PMP: 169. See for an analysis of the virtues or 'personal qualities' that might follow from Adorno's practical philosophy: Finlayson 2002: 7.
29. PMP: 169–70.
30. See also Freyenhagen 2013: 168–9.
31. AE: 155.

32. ND: 365.
33. PMP: 97.
34. ND: 185–6.
35. ND: 203.
36. ND: 17–18.
37. M: 116–17.
38. ND: 366.
39. PMP: 145. See also Gerhardt 2006: 172. See for an emphasis on the animality of this impulse and its contrast with 'bourgeois coldness': Freyenhagen 2008: 108.
40. See also Bernstein 2001: 386.
41. MM: 105 n1.
42. MM: 105.
43. See for example BM: 69, 149.
44. Peter Dews is one of the few authors in the English-speaking academic world who notices this: 'it is clear that Adorno's account of the 'addendum' has been deeply influenced by Schopenhauer's critique of Kant's rationalism, and his conception of compassion (*Mitleid*) as the wellspring of ethical action' (Dews 2008: 205). See also Schweppenhäuser 2004: 333–5.
45. See also Früchtl 1991: 38–9.
46. See also Zuidervaart 2007: 61.
47. Spierling 1985:16. ['Only with closed eyes can direct perceptions of existential experiences of pain be thought ["philosophized"] away with help of secondary concepts. Schopenhauer tries to put a stop to philosophical justifications of suffering. He "blocks" philosophy by positioning corporeal pain in its way.' – My translation.]
48. ND: 203.
49. See also Freyenhagen 2013:143.
50. PMP: 9.
51. See for a discussion of the mediated nature of the moral addendum: Cook 2011: 127. See on the nature of our impulses of solidarity also: Menke 2006: 77. See for an Aristotelian understanding of our bodily responses to specific situations: Freyenhagen 2013: 250–1. Zuidervaart argues that suffering bears an intrinsic normative value, in Adorno's view (Zuidervaart 2007: 61). He himself, however, claims that suffering always needs to be interpreted and embedded in theory in order to function as part of a moral way of thinking (see Zuidervaart 2007: 68; Zuidervaart 1991: 306). Zuidervaart observes that feelings of compassion are often used to rationalize certain (political) goals and that Adorno therefore should embed these feelings in a moral theory as well. In this chapter, however, I argue that Adorno precisely refers to the way compassion is often used for political gain to defend the idea that it should *not* be rationalized.
52. Scarry 1985: 51, 54–5.
53. Améry himself rejects attempts to explain the evil of Nazi Germany, criticizing 'the sophisticated speculations about the dialectics of enlightenment' for telling us nothing about the 'singular and irreducible' nature of evil, characterized by a 'total inner logic' and an 'accursed rationality' (Améry viii). Instead, he claims that torture formed the essence of the Third Reich (Améry 1980: 24).
54. Améry 1980: 40.
55. Améry 1980: 33.

56. Valéry 1980: 33.
57. Vetlesen 2009: 73.
58. Vetlesen 2009: 52.
59. Scarry 1985: 5.
60. Améry 1980: 9.
61. NK: 227.
62. See M: 117–18.
63. See also Schweppenhäuser 2004: 346.
64. AT: 18.
65. See also Cook 2011: 127.
66. M: 104.
67. ND: 365.
68. M: 116.
69. ND: 299. See also Früchtl 1993.
70. NK: 237.
71. NK: 237 Adorno may also have had Marx's claim in mind that 'political economy knows the worker only as a working-animal – as a beast reduced to the strictest bodily needs' (Marx 1988: 29).
72. Améry 1980: xi.
73. See also Freyenhagen 2013: 197.
74. See for an excellent analysis of this 'ethics of resistance': Freyenhagen 2013: 162–6.
75. See also ND: 41.
76. ND: 287.
77. See also Adorno 1971: 144.
78. See also Freyenhagen 2013: 95–100.
79. See also Freyenhagen 2013: 194–5.
80. This observation returns in the social antinomy embodied by humanitarian aid: on the one hand, this kind of aid does not structurally change the conditions under which people suffer and may even affirm these conditions. On the other hand, humanitarian aid may be the only way to do something about suffering within a social whole that does not allow structural changes to be made, at least not in the foreseeable future.

9 The Road to Salvation

1. See Zenith 2006: xiii.
2. Zenith 2006: xx.
3. Pessoa 2006: 68.
4. Pessoa 2006: 71.
5. Young 1987: 146.
6. WWR-I: 390.
7. A passage like the following from the *Mundaka Upanishad* describes a similar experience: 'a man whose mind wanders among desires, and is longing for objects of desire, goes again to life and death according to his desires. But he who possesses the End of all longing, and whose self has found fulfilment, even in this life his desire will fade away' (*The Upanishads* 1965: 81). The radically pessimistic nature of the methods of self-denial that Schopenhauer

advocates, however, should not be underestimated. In his study of Schopenhauer and Eastern forms of thought, Ray Singh insightfully argues that the denial that Schopenhauer defends is much more radical, because it is based on a much more pessimistic (and, in Raj Singh's view, simplistic) evaluation of the world than the denial defended by Vedanta and Buddhism (Raj Singh 2007:105–7). See also Cooper 2012; Barua (and others): 2013.

8. WWR-I: 410.
9. WWR-I: 408–9.
10. WWR-I: 409.
11. WWR-II: 325–6.
12. WWR-II: 610–11. See also Raj Singh 2007: 65.
13. WWR-II: 612.
14. WWR-II: 641.
15. Certain aspects of these observations remind one of Wittgenstein's ladder-metaphor in *Tractatus Logico-Philosophicus*, according to which the ladder provided by the text itself is thrown away once Wittgenstein has reached the point from which he is able to show that this text cannot say what it means. As several commentators have argued, Schopenhauer's philosophy, especially its mystical aspects and its focus on silence, had a profound influence on Wittgenstein's early philosophy. See for example Janaway 1999c: 317–42; Magee 1983: 310–39; Hannan 2009: 141; Schroeder 2012. Famously, Wittgenstein states in a Schopenhauerian manner: 'There is indeed the inexpressible. This shows itself; it is the mystical' (Wittgenstein 2001: § 6.522).
16. See also Hannan 2009: 140–1.
17. WWR-I: 198–9.
18. WWR-I: 383.
19. See also Guyer 2009: 19.
20. WWR-I: 200.
21. WWR-II: 368.
22. See for a defence of the first view Magee 1983: 239; and see for the second interpretation Janaway 1996: 29.
23. WWR-I: 175.
24. See WWR-II: 374.
25. See WWR-II: 369.
26. WWR-II: 374.
27. See WWR-II: 374.
28. WWR-I: 170.
29. See WWR-II: 364.
30. WWR-II: 364.
31. See WWR-II: 366.
32. WWR-I: 179.
33. WWR-I: 198–9.
34. See WWR-II: 367.
35. WWR-II: 363.
36. WWR-I: 197.
37. WWR-I: 252.
38. WWR-I: 254.
39. WWR-I: 253.

40. WWR-I: 253.
41. See Vandenabeele 2009: 50; Guyer 2009: 21.
42. WWR-I: 256.
43. WWR-I: 263.
44. WWR-I: 260.
45. WWR-I: 262.
46. WWR-I: 263.
47. WWR-I: 202.
48. WWR-II: 450.
49. WWR-I: 202.
50. See also Vandenabeele 2009: 45; Guyer 1996: 129; Foster 1996: 140.WWR-I: 220.
51. WWR-I: 220. See also Foster 1996: 140. It could perhaps be argued that the paintings of Francis Bacon, whom I briefly discussed in Chapter 2, could, within Schopenhauer's aesthetic theory, be positioned 'in between' his analyses of tragedy and music. On the one hand, these paintings force us to *realize* that we are flesh and, to a certain extent, subject to the same desires and forces that pull apart the flesh of the beings that Bacon paints. On the other hand, there is a sense of beauty in Bacon's paintings that could be characterized as *sublime*: if we violently tear ourselves away, *as individuals*, from the flesh his paintings depict, we may experience a kinship with this same flesh and the beautiful forms, shapes, colours and movements of its depictions.
52. WWR-II: 363.
53. WWR-I: 379.
54. BM: 210.
55. BM: 212.
56. WWR-I: 368.
57. WWR-I: 380.
58. BM: 147.
59. WWR-II: 608.
60. DS: 304.
61. WWR-I: 373.
62. WWR-I: 380.
63. WWR-I: 381.
64. WWR-I: 391.
65. WWR-I: 383.
66. WWR-I: 397.
67. WWR-I: 382.
68. In a peculiar passage, Schopenhauer for example argues that the beauty of light, reflection and colours is constituted by a 'mere sensation of the retina's affection' that, because it is a sensation 'wholly free from pain and pleasure', results in 'pure knowledge'. This means that he is not blind to the observation that sensation has to play a role in aesthetic enjoyment (WWR-II: 375). This passage is peculiar, because Schopenhauer here explicitly equates 'pure knowing' with 'mere sensation' and, in turn, with 'enjoyment'. Sensation *itself* here seems to be the source of beauty and enjoyment, a claim that conflicts acutely with his focus on Platonic Ideas. Interestingly,

this passage reminds one of the beginning of Aristotle's *Metaphysics*, with which Schopenhauer must have been familiar: 'By nature, all men long to know. An indication is their delight in the senses. For these, quite apart from their utility, are intrinsically delightful, and that through the eyes more than the others. For it is not only with a view to action but also when we have no intention to do anything that we choose, so to speak, sight rather than all the others. And the reason for this is that sight is the sense that especially produces cognition in us and reveals many distinguishing features of things' (Aristotle 1998: 4).

69. WWR-II: 364.
70. WWR-I: 253.
71. WWR-I: 253
72. WWR-II: 507.
73. WWR-II: 573.
74. WWRI: 301.
75. WWRI: 288.
76. WWRI: 288, 301.
77. WWRI: 288.
78. WWR-I: 411.
79. See also Atwell 1995: 184; Atwell 1990: 185–6.
80. WWR-I: 202.
81. Janaway 1997: 94–5.
82. Janaway 1999c: 284.
83. Lukács 1980: 188.
84. WWR-I: xii. Schopenhauer makes this claim at several places, see also WN: 374.
85. See also Janaway 1999b: 287.
86. See for example Magee 1983: 242.
87. As quoted in Magee 1983: 409.
88. Simmel 1991: 59. See also Dews 2008: 123.
89. Horkheimer 1974b: 72–3.
90. See Magee 1983: 350–417; Janaway 1997: 101; Vandenabeele 2012: 7. Jack Kerouac mentions Schopenhauer in *On the Road* as well (see Kerouac 1957: 6).
91. See Tolstoy 2008: 37–8.
92. Maas 2010: 774–7.
93. Büttner 2002: 115.
94. As quoted in Büttner 2002: 115.
95. As described in Young 2009: 158–60.
96. Kierkegaard 1988. See for this interpretation: Mannion 2003: 240.
97. Young 2009: 157. The phrase 'four noble truths' is, of course, a reference to the four noble truths that constitute Buddhism: (1)Our existence is defined by suffering; (2) This suffering is caused by the nature of the world, which is striving; (3) It is possible to overcome this state of suffering and reach an experience of nothingness and bliss; (4) This can be done by following several paths and by performing several practices. See also Janaway 1997: 94.
98. WWR-I: 404.
99. Kierkegaard 1983: 80. See on this topic also: Kierkegaard 1992: 54–6.

100. WWR-II: 408.
101. In his *Journals and Papers* Kierkegaard himself expressed an ambivalent but in places personal admiration for Schopenhauer. In his journal of 1854, for example, he writes: 'A.S. is unquestionably an important writer; he has interested me very much and I am astonished to find an author who, in spite of complete disagreement, touches me at so many points', noticing: 'Curiously enough I am called S.A. and we probably stand in an inverse relation to one another' (Kierkegaard 1967–78: § 4.26, XI.1 A 144).
102. Mannion 2003: 281.
103. Mannion 2003: 270.
104. Mannion 2003: 273.
105. Mannion 2003: 237.
106. WWR-I: 405.
107. WWR-I: 404.
108. See for example Schopenhauer 2000b: 210–11.
109. Schopenhauer 2000c: 394
110. Schopenhauer 2000c: 394.
111. DS: 301.
112. Mannion 2003: 41–52.
113. WWR-II: 580.
114. Horkheimer 1974b: 83.

10 *Rien Faire Comme une Bête*

1. Proust 1992: 294.
2. Proust 1992: 305.
3. Proust 1992: 437.
4. Proust 1992: 437.
5. Proust 1992: 528.
6. M: 104.
7. M: 105.
8. M: 104.
9. M: 104.
10. ND: 366–7.
11. ND: 362.
12. M: 141.
13. ND: 361.
14. ND: 377–8. Adorno's reference to the 'awakening of genius' clearly refers to the following passage: 'Awakened to life out of the night of unconsciousness, the will finds itself as an individual in an endless and boundless world, among innumerable individuals, all striving, suffering, and erring; and, as if through a troubled dream, it hurries back to the old unconsciousness' (WWR-II: 573).
15. Adorno makes a similar point in *Negative Dialectics* (see ND: 325–6). See also Früchtl 1991: 37.
16. ND: 407.
17. See also Bernstein 2001: 426.
18. M: 140.

19. M: 140.
20. M: 140.
21. See M: 140.
22. M: 140.
23. M: 141.
24. See M: 141.
25. M: 142.
26. Proust 1992: 115.
27. M: 145.
28. See also Freyenhagen 2013: 226–7.
29. WWR-II: 394.
30. See Finlayson 2009 : 15.
31. See also Dews 2008: 205.
32. See also Finlayson 2009: 14.
33. AT: 311.
34. AT: 311.
35. ND: 378.
36. ND: 378.
37. ND: 378.
38. See MM: 155n.
39. MM: 157.
40. MM: 228.
41. Proust 1992: 240.
42. WWR-I: 260.
43. MM: 175.
44. Adorno 2001a : 191–2.
45. Adorno 2001a : 187.
46. See Büttner 2002: 119.
47. UE: 289. It could even be argued that whereas the two protagonists of Beckett's *Waiting for Godot* (1987) still find solace in a Schopenhauerian form of compassion with each other, the protagonists of *Endgame* have left this state behind and are in a process of denying both their selves and their bodies. From an Adornian point of view, the difference between the Schopenhauerian traces in these plays can be interpreted as mirroring the historical decline of society.
48. M: 117.
49. See also Raponi 2003.
50. As quoted in McDonald 2009: xv.
51. UE: 294.
52. AT: 260.
53. AT: 153–4.
54. In *Minima Moralia* Adorno makes this same point by arguing that speech, conversation and communication have been permeated and pathologized by social categories to such an extent that verbal forms of contact have become meaningless gestures (MM: 90).
55. AT: 226.
56. Adorno 1984: 155–6.
57. PMM: 49.
58. NK: 237.
59. AT: 258.

60. PMM: 92.
61. M: 118.
62. M: 118.
63. See M: 117–18.
64. UE: 261.
65. UE: 286.
66. See M: 116.
67. M: 11
68. ND: 262–3.
69. PMM: 30.
70. AT: 135–6.
71. See also Finlayson 2009: 8.
72. AT: 258.
73. PMM: 95.
74. As quoted in Bowie 2004: 267. See also Zuidervaart 1991: 128.
75. Espen Hammer 2006: 105.
76. Adorno 2003d: 306.
77. Adorno 2003d: 331.
78. PMM: 95–6.
79. AT: 346.
80. DS: 300.
81. ND: 403. Translation amended by me: 'philosophem' has been changed into 'philosopheme'.
82. Marx 1990: 169.
83. ND: 284.
84. ND: 262.
85. Habermas 1984; Honneth 1995.
86. MM: 23.
87. MM: 157.
88. ND: 244.
89. See also Leppert 2005: 93.
90. ND: 203–4.
91. See ND: 185; DE 156.
92. See also Cook 2011: 123; Jarvis 2004: 97; Jarvis 2007: 263.
93. MM: 228.
94. PMP: 169–70.
95. See ND: 321; DE: 36–7.
96. ND: 191.
97. Dews 2008: 204–5.
98. DE: 214.
99. ND: 207.
100. See also Cook 2011: 112.
101. AT: 15.

11 Conclusion

1. See for an interesting comparison of Schopenhauer and Coetzee's ideas on animal ethics Muratori 2008.
2. Coetzee 1999: 65.

3. Coetzee 1999: 26.
4. Singer 1999: 90.
5. Singer 1999: 88–9.
6. As quoted in New York Times 1987.
7. ND: 404.
8. Adorno even observes in *Negative Dialectics*: 'according to every psychological insight even Hitler and his monsters were slaves to their early childhood, products of mental mutilation' (ND: 264).

Bibliography

Works by Adorno

(1955) *The Authoritarian Personality (Studies in Prejudice)* (New York: Harper and Brothers) [with M. Horkheimer, R. Nevitt Sanford, D.J. Levinson, E. Frenkel-Brunswik et al].

(1971) 'Erziehung zur Mündigkeit' in *Erziehung zur Mündigkeit* (Frankfurt: Suhrkamp).

(1973) *Negative Dialectics*, transl. E.B. Ashton (New York: Continuum).

(1974) *Minima Moralia: Reflections from Damaged Life*, transl. E. Jephcott (London: Verso).

(1984) 'The Essay as Form', trans. B. Hullot-Kentor, F. Will. *New German Critique*, 32, 151–71.

(1985) *Against Epistemology: A Metacritique; Studies in Husserl and the Phenomenological Antinomies*, transl. W. Domingo (Cambridge: The MIT Press).

(1991) 'Extorted Reconciliation: On Georg Lukács' *Realism in Our Time*' in *Notes to Literature. Volume 1*, ed. R. Tiedemann, transl. S.W. Nicholsen (New York: Columbia University Press).

(1993) *Hegel: Three Studies*, transl. S. Weber Nicholsen (Cambridge, MS: The MIT Press).

(1997) *Aesthetic Theory*, transl. R. Hullot-Kentor (Minneapolis, MN: University of Minnesota Press).

(1998a) 'On Subject and Object' in *Critical Models. Interventions and Catchwords*, transl. H.W. Pickford (New York: Columbia University Press).

(1998b) 'Sexual Taboos and Law Today' in *Critical Models*, transl. H.W. Pickford (New York: Columbia University Press).

(1998c) 'Why still Philosophy' in *Critical Models*, transl. H.W. Pickford (New York: Columbia University Press).

(2000a) *Metaphysics – Concepts and Problems: Lectures 1965*, ed. R. Tiedemann, transl. E. Jephcott (Cambridge: Polity Press).

(2000b) *Problems of Moral Philosophy – Lectures 1963*, ed. T. Schröder, transl. R. Livingstone (Cambridge: Polity Press).

(2001a) 'Free Time' in *The Culture Industry*, ed. J. Bernstein, transl. G. Finlayson, N. Walker (New York, NY).

(2001b) 'The Schema of Mass Culture' in *The Culture Industry*, ed. J. Bernstein, transl. A.G. Rabinbach (New York, NY).

(2002) *Dialectic of Enlightenment; Philosophical Fragments*, transl. E. Jephcott (Stanford: Stanford University Press).

(2003a) 'Cultural Criticism and Society' in *Can One Live after Auschwitz?*, ed. R. Tiedemann (Stanford: Stanford University Press).

(2003b) 'Education after Auschwitz' in *Can One Live after Auschwitz?*, ed. R. Tiedeman, transl. Henry W. Pickford (Stanford: Stanford University Press).

(2003c) 'Notes on Kafka' in *Can One Live after Auschwitz?*, ed. R. Tiedemann, transl. S. Weber, S. Weber Nicholsen (Stanford: Stanford University Press).

(2003d) 'Schubert' in *Can One Live after Auschwitz?*, ed. R. Tiedemann, transl. R. Livingstone (Stanford: Stanford University Press).

(2003e) 'The Meaning of Working through the Past' in *Can One Live after Auschwitz?*, ed. R. Tiedemann, transl. H.W. Pickford (Stanford: Stanford University Press).

(2003f) 'Trying to Understand *Endgame*' in *Can One Live after Auschwitz?*, ed. R. Tiedemann, transl. S. Weber Nicholsen (Stanford: Stanford University Press).

(2006) *History and Freedom: Lectures 1964–1965*, ed. R. Tiedemann, transl. R. Livingstone (Cambridge: Polity Press).

(2007) *Philosophy of Modern Music*, transl. A.G. Mitchell, W.V. Blomster (London: Continuum).

(2008) *Lectures on Negative Dialectics: Fragments of a Lecture Course 1965/1966*, ed. R. Tiedemann, transl. R. Livingstone (Cambridge: Polity Press).

(2009) *The Jargon of Authenticity*, transl. K. Tarnowski, F. Will (New York: Routledge).

Works by Schopenhauer

(1960) *Essay on the Freedom of the Will*, transl. K. Kolenda (New York: Dover Publications).

(1969) *The World as Will and Representation* [two volumes], transl. E.F.J. Payne (New York: Dover Publications).

(1985) *Metaphysik der Sitten (Philosophische Vorlesungen Teil IV)*, ed. V. Spierling (München: Piper Verlag).

(1987) *Reisetagebücher* (Zürich: Haffmans Verlag).

(1995) *On the Basis of Morality*, transl. E.F.J. Payne (Indianapolis: Hacket Publishing).

(2000a) 'Additional Remarks on the Doctrine of the Suffering of the World' in *Parerga and Paralipomena. Volume II*, transl. E.F.J. Payne (Oxford: Clarendon Press).

(2000b) 'On Ethics' in *Parerga and Paralipomena. Volume II*, transl. E.F.J. Payne (Oxford: Clarendon Press).

(2000c) 'On Religion' in *Parerga and Paralipomena. Volume II*, transl. E.F.J. Payne (Oxford: Clarendon Press).

(2000d) 'On Suicide' in *Parerga and Paralipomena. Volume II*, transl. E.F.J. Payne (Oxford: Clarendon Press).

(2000e) 'On Women' in *Parerga and Paralipomena. Volume II*, transl. E.F.J. Payne (Oxford: Clarendon Press).

(2000e) 'Psychological Remarks' in *Parerga and Paralipomena. Volume II*, transl. E.F.J. Payne (Oxford: Clarendon Press).

(2007a) *On the Fourfold Root of the Principle of Sufficient Reason*, transl. Mme. K. Hillebrand (New York: Cosimo Classics).

(2007b) *On the Will in Nature*, transl. Mme. K. Hillebrand (New York: Cosimo Classics).

Works by other authors

Améry, J. (1980) *At the Mind's Limits: Contemplations by a Survivor on Auschwitz and Its Realities*, transl. S. Rosenfeld, S.P. Rosenfeld (Indianapolis: Indiana University Press).

Aristotle (1998) *Metaphysics*, transl. H. Lawson-Tancred (London: Penguin).

Atwell, J.E. (1990) *Schopenhauer: The Human Character* (Philadelphia: Temple University Press).

—— (1995) *Schopenhauer on the Character of the World; The Metaphysics of Will* (Berkeley: University of California Press).

Atzert, S. (2012) 'Schopenhauer and Freud' in B. Vandenabeele (ed.) *A Companion to Schopenhauer* (Oxford: Blackwell Publishing).

Barua, A., Gerhard, M., Kossler, M. (eds) (2013) *Understanding Schopenhauer Through the Prism of Indian Culture* (Berlin: De Gruyter).

Beckett, S. (1987) *Waiting for Godot* (Stuttgart: Philipp Reklam).

—— (2009) *Endgame* (London: Faber and Faber).

Benhabib, S. (1986) *Critique, Norm, and Utopia; a Study of the Foundations of Critical Theory* (New York: Columbia University Press).

Bernstein, J.M. (2001) *Adorno: Disenchantment and Ethics* (Cambridge: Cambridge University Press).

Bishop, P. (2003) 'Social Critique and Aesthetics in Schopenhauer', *History of European Ideas*, 29(4), 411–35.

Blondel, E. (1991) *Nietzsche: The Body and Culture. Philosophy as a Philological Genealogy*, transl. S. Hand (London: The Athlone Press).

Bowie, A. (2004) 'Adorno, Heidegger, and the Meaning of Music' in T. Huhn (ed.) *The Cambridge Companion to Adorno* (Cambridge: Cambridge University Press).

Brink, B. van den (1997) 'Gesellschaftstheorie und Übertreibungskunst (Für eine alternative Lesart der "Dialektik der Aufklärung"', *Neue Rundschau*, 108, 37–59.

Butler, J. (1998) 'Gender and Performance: Selections from *Gender Trouble*' in D. Welton (ed.) *Body and Flesh: A Philosophical Reader* (Malden, MA: Blackwell).

Büttner, G. (2002) 'Schopenhauer's Recommendations to Beckett' in A. Moorjani, C. Veit (eds) *Samuel Beckett Today/Aujourd'hui* (Amsterdam/New York: Editions Rodopi).

Came, D. (2012) 'Schopenhauer on the Metaphysics of Art and Morality' in B. Vandenabeele (ed.) *A Companion to Schopenhauer* (Oxford: Blackwell Publishing).

Cartwright, D.E. (1981) 'Scheler's Criticisms of Schopenhauer's Theory of "Mitleid", *Jahrbuch der Schopenhauer-Gesellschaft*, 62, 144–52.

—— (1989) 'Schopenhauer as Moral Philosopher: Towards the Actuality of his Ethics', *Jahrbuch der Schopenhauer-Gesellschaft*, 70, 54–65.

—— (2009) 'Compassion and Solidarity with Sufferers: the Metaphysics of Mitleid' in A. Neil, C. Janaway (eds) *Better Consciousness: Schopenhauer's Philosophy of Value* (Chisester: Wiley-Blackwell).

Clendinnen, I. (2002) *Reading the Holocaust* (Cambridge: Cambridge University Press).

Coetzee, J.M. [et al] (1999) *The Lives of Animals*, ed. Amy Gutman (Princeton, NJ: Princeton University Press).

—— (2000) *Disgrace* (London: Vintage).

Cook, D. (2011) *Adorno on Nature* (Durham: Acumen).

Cooper, D.E. (2012) 'Schopenhauer and Indian Philosophy' in B. Vandenabeele (ed.) *A Companion to Schopenhauer* (Oxford: Blackwell Publishing).

Cornell, D. (1987) 'The Ethical Message of Negative Dialectics', *Social Concept*, 4(1), 3–38.

Damasio, A. (2005) *Descartes' Error: Emotion, Reason, and the Human Brain* (New York: Harper Collins).

Deleuze, G. (2005) *Francis Bacon: The Logic of Sensation*, transl. D.W. Smith (London: Continuum).

Dews, P. (2008) *The Idea of Evil* (Malden, MA: Blackwell Publishing).

Dörflinger, B. (2002) 'Schopenhauers Philosophie des Leibes', *Jahrbuch der Schopenhauer-Gesellschaft*, 83, 43–85.

Dörpinghaus, A. (2000) 'Der Leib als Schlüssel zur Welt. Zur Bedeutung und Funktion des Leibes in der Philosophie A. Schopenhauers', *Jahrbuch der Schopenhauer-Gesellschaft*, 81, 15–31.

Dowd, G. (2009) 'Apprenticeship, Philosophy, and the "Secret Pressures of the Work of Art" in Deleuze, Beckett, Proust and Ruiz; or Remaking the *Recherche*' in M. Bryden, M. Topping (eds) *Beckett's Proust/Deleuze's Proust* (New York: Palgrave Macmillan).

Einstein, A. (1997) 'My Credo' in Robert N. Goldman (ed.) *Einstein's God: Albert Einstein's Quest as a Scientist and as a Jew to Replace a Forsaken God* (Joyce Aronson Inc.: Northvale, New Jersey).

Finlayson, J.G. (2002) 'Adorno on the Ethical and the Ineffable', *European Journal of Philosophy*, 10(1), 1–25.

—— (2009) 'The Work of Art and the Promise of Happiness in Adorno', *World Pictures*, 3.

Foster, C. (1996) 'Schopenhauer and Aesthetic Recognition' in D. Jacquette (ed.) *Schopenhauer, Philosophy, and the Arts* (Cambridge: Cambridge University Press).

Foucault, M. (1994) 'Nietzsche, Freud, Marx' in *Aesthetics, Method, and Epistemology*, transl. R. Hurley, ed. J.D. Faubion (New York: The New Press).

—— (1990) *The Use of Pleasure: The History of Sexuality Volume 2*, transl. R. Hurley (London: Penguin Books).

—— (1998a) *The Will to Knowledge: The History of Sexuality Volume 1*, transl. R. Hurley (London: Penguin Books).

—— (1998b) *The Care of the Self: The History of Sexuality Volume 3*, transl. R. Hurley (London: Penguin Books).

Freud, S. (1961) *Civilization and its Discontents*, transl. James Strachey (New York, NY: WW. Norton & Company).

Freyenhagen, F. (2006) 'Adorno's Negative Dialectics of Freedom', *Philosophy and Social Criticism*, 32(3), 429–40.

—— (2008) 'Moral Philosophy' in Deborah Cook (ed.) *Theodor Adorno: Key Concepts* (Stocksfield: Acumen).

—— (2013) *Adorno's Practical Philosophy: Living Less Wrongly* (Cambridge: Cambridge University Press).

Früchtl, J. (1991) '"Moral begründen ist schwer." Die Rolle der Mitleidsethik bei Adorno und Habermas', *Jahrbuch der Schopenhauer-Gesellschaft*, 72, 36–44.

—— (1993) '"Leben wie ein gutes Tier": Ethik Zwischen Mitleid und Diskurs', *Deutsche Zeitung für Philosophie*, 41(6), 981–94.

Gardner, S. (1999) 'Schopenhauer, Will, and the Unconscious' in C. Janaway (ed.) *The Cambridge Companion to Schopenhauer* (Cambridge: Cambridge University Press).

Gerhardt, C. (2006) 'The Ethics of Animals in Adorno and Kafka', *New German Critique*, 97, 159–78.

Gimmel, J. (2011) 'Metaphysische Erfahrung und Verzweiflung', *Jahrbuch der Schopenhauer-Gesellschaft*, 92, 135–59.

Guyer, P. (1996) 'Pleasure and Knowledge in Schopenhauer's Aesthetics' in D. Jacquette (ed.) *Schopenhauer, Philosophy, and the Arts* (Cambridge: Cambridge University Press).
—— (1999) 'Schopenhauer, Kant, and the Methods of Philosophy' in C. Janaway (ed.) *The Cambridge Companion to Schopenhauer* (Cambridge: Cambridge University Press).
—— (2009) 'Back to Truth: Knowledge and Pleasure in the Aesthetics of Schopenhauer' in A. Neil, C. Janaway (eds) *Better Consciousness: Schopenhauer's Philosophy of Value* (Chisester: Wiley-Blackwell).
Habermas, J. (1984) *The Theory of Communicative Action. Volume One: reason and the Rationalization of Society*, transl. T. McCarthy (Boston: Beacon Press)
—— (1990) 'The Entwinement of Myth and Enlightenment: Max Horkheimer and Theodor W. Adorno' in *The Philosophical Discourse of Modernity*, transl. Frederick G. Lawrence (Cambridge, MA: Cambridge University Press).
Hamington, M. (2004) *Embodied Care: Jane Addams, Maurice Merleau-Ponty, and Feminist Ethics* (Chicago, IL: University of Illinois Press).
Hammer, E. (2006) *Adorno and the Political* (London: Routledge).
Hannan, B. (2009) *The Riddle of the World: A Reconsideration of Schopenhauer's Philosophy* (Oxford: Oxford University Press).
Hearfield, C. (2004) *Adorno and the Modern Ethos of Freedom* (Hampshire: Ashgate).
Hegel, G.W.F. (1977) *Phenomenology of Spirit*, transl. A.V. Miller (Oxford: Oxford University Press).
Herron, T. (2005) 'The Dog Man; Becoming Animal in Coetzee's Disgrace', *Twentieth-Century Literature*, 51(4), 467–90.
Hobbes, T. (1983) *De Cive*, ed. H. Warrender (Oxford: Oxford University Press).
Honneth, A. (1995) *The Struggle for Recognition: The Moral Grammar of Social Conflicts*, transl. J. Anderson (Cambridge: Polity Press).
—— (2000) 'Über die Möglichkeit einer erschliessenden Gesellschaftskritik; Die "Dialektik der Aufklärung" im Horizont gegenwärtiger Debatten über Sozialkritik' in *Das Andere der Gerechtigkeit: Aufsätze zur praktischen Philosophie* (Frankfurt/M: Surhkamp).
Horkheimer, M. (1955) 'Schopenhauer und die Gesellschaft', *Jahrbuch der Schopenhauer-Gesellschaft*, 36, 49–57.
—— (1961) 'Die Aktualität Schopenhauers' in *Jahrbuch der Schopenhauer-Gesellschaft*, 42, 12–25.
—— (1972) 'Materialism and Metaphysics' in *Critical Theory: Selected Essays*, transl. M.J. O'Connell (New York: The Seabury Press).
—— (1974a) *Eclipse of Reason* (London: Continuum).
—— (1974b) 'Schopenhauer Today' in *Critique of Instrumental Reason*, transl. M.J. O'Connell (New York: The Seabury Press).
Houellebecq, M. (2004) 'Gesprek met Martin de Haan' in M. de Haan (ed.) *De Koude Revolutie. Confrontaties en Bespiegelingen* (Amsterdam: Uitgeverij De Arbeiderspers).
Hume, D. (1983) *An Enquiry Concerning the Principles of Morals* (Indianapolis, IN: Hackett Publishing Company).
—— (2003) *A Treatise of Human Nature* (New York: Dover Publications).
Hutcheson, F. (2002) *An Essay on the Nature and Conducts of the Passions and Affections, with Illustrations on the Moral Sense*, ed. A. Garrett (Indianapolis: Liberty Fund).

Janaway, C. (1996) 'Knowledge and Tranquility: Schopenhauer on the Value of Art' in D. Jacquette (ed.) *Schopenhauer, Philosophy, and the Arts* (Cambridge, Cambridge University Press).
—— (1997) *Schopenhauer* (Oxford: Oxford University Press).
—— (1999a) 'Introduction' in C. Janaway (ed.) *The Cambridge Companion to Schopenhauer* (Cambridge: Cambridge University Press).
—— (1999b) 'Schopenhauer's Pessimism' in C. Janaway (ed.) *The Cambridge Companion to Schopenhauer* (Cambridge: Cambridge University Press).
—— (1999c) *Self and World in Schopenhauer's Philosophy* (Oxford: Oxford University Press).
Jarvis, S. (2004) 'Adorno, Marx, Materialism' in T. Huhn (ed.) *The Cambridge Companion to Adorno* (Cambridge: Cambridge University Press).
—— (2007) 'The Coastline of Experience: Materialism and Metaphysics in Adorno' in S. Jarvis (ed.) *Theodor W. Adorno – Volume III – Critical Evaluations in Cultural Theory* (Abingdon: Routledge).
Jay, M. (1973) *The Dialectical Imagination: A History of the Frankfurt School and the Institute of Social Research* (Berkeley: University of California Press).
Jordan, J. (2001) 'The Unconscious' in R. Bales (ed.) *The Cambridge Companion to Proust* (Cambridge: Cambridge University Press).
Jordan, N. (2009) 'Schopenhauer's Politics: Ethics, Jurisprudence and the State' in A. Neil, C. Janaway (eds) *Better Consciousness: Schopenhauer's Philosophy of Value* (Chisester: Wiley-Blackwell).
Jütten, T. (2012) 'Adorno on Kant, Freedom and Determinism', *European Journal of Philosophy*, 20(4), 548–74.
Kafka, F. (2007) *In the Penal Colony*, transl. Michael Hofman (London: Penguin Books).
Kant, I. (1977) *Prolegomena to Any Future Metaphysics*, transl. James W. Ellington (Cambridge, IN: Hackett Publishing).
—— (1999) 'An Answer to the Question: What is enlightenment?' in *Practical Philosophy*, transl. ed. M.J. Gregor (Cambridge: Cambridge University Press).
—— (2003) *Critique of Pure Reason*, transl. J.M.D. Meiklejohn (Mineola, NY: Dover Publications).
—— (2004) *Critique of Practical Reason*, transl. T.K. Abbott (Mineola, NY: Dover Publications).
—— (2011) *Groundwork of the Metaphysics of Morals. A German-English Edition*, transl. M. Gregor (Cambridge: Cambridge University Press).
Kerouac, J. (1957) *On the Road* (New York: Penguin Books).
Kierkegaard, S. (1967–78) *Journals and Papers*, 7 volumes, ed. transl. Howard V. Hong, E.H. Hong (Princeton NJ: Princeton University Press).
—— (1983) *Fear and Trembling; Repetition*, ed. transl. H.V. Hong, E.H. Hong (Princeton NJ: Princeton University Press).
—— (1988) *Stages on Life's Way. Studies by Various Persons*, ed. transl. H.V. Hong, E.H. Hong (Princeton NJ: Princeton University Press).
—— (1992) *Concluding Unscientific Postscript to Philosophical Fragments*, ed. transl. H.V. Hong, E.H. Hong (Princeton NJ: Princeton University Press).
Korsgaard, C. (1996) *The Sources of Normativity* (Cambridge: Cambridge University Press).
—— (2006) 'Morality and the Distinctiveness of Human Action' in F. de Waal, *Primates and Philosophers: How Morality Evolved*, ed. S. Macedo, J. Ober (Princeton: Princeton University Press).

—— (2008) 'From Duty and for the Sake of the Noble: Kant and Aristotle on Morally Good Action' in *The Constitution of Agency* (Oxford: Oxford University Press).
—— (2009) *Self-Constitution: Agency, Identity, and Integrity* (Cambridge: Cambridge University Press).
Leder, D. (1998) 'A Tale of Two Bodies: The Cartesian Corpse and the Lived Body' in D. Welton (ed.) *Body and Flesh: A Philosophical Reader* (Malden, MA: Blackwell).
Lee, L.Y. (2005) *Dialectics of the Body: Corporeality in the Philosophy of T.W. Adorno* (New York: Routledge).
Leibniz, G.W. (2007) 'Essays on the Justice of God and the Freedom of Man in the Origin of Evil' in *Theodicy*, ed. A. Farrer, transl. E.M. Huggard (Charleston, SC: BiblioBazaar).
Leppert, R. (2005) 'Music "Pushed to the Edge of Existence" (Adorno, Listening, and the Question of Hope)', *Cultural Critique*, 60, 92–133.
Levin, D.M. (1999) 'The Ontological Dimension of Embodiment: Heidegger's Thinking of Being' in D. Welton (ed.) *The Body: Classic and Contemporary Readings* (Malden, MA: Blackwell).
Lukács, G. (1968) *History and Class Consciousness: Studies in Marxist Dialectics*, transl. R. Livingstone (Cambridge, MS: The MIT Press).
—— (1980) 'The Bourgeois Irrationalism of Schopenhauer's Metaphysics' in M. Fox (ed.) *Schopenhauer: His Philosophical Achievement* (Sussex: The Harvester Press).
—— (1988) *The Theory of the Novel: A Historico-Philosophical Essay on the Forms of Great Epic Literature*, transl. A. Bostock (London: The Merlin Press).
Maas, N. (2010) *Gerard Reve. Kroniek van een Schuldig Leven. Deel 2 – De 'Rampjaren' (1962 – 1975)* (Amsterdam: G.A. van Oorschot).
Magee, B. (1983) *The Philosophy of Schopenhauer* (Oxford: Clarendon Press).
Mannion, G. (2003) *Schopenhauer, Religion and Morality: The Humble Path to Ethics* (Hants: Ashgate).
Marcuse, H. (1974) *Eros and Civilization: A Philosophical Inquiry into Freud* (Boston: Beacon Press).
Marx, K. (1988) *Economic and Philosophic Manuscripts of 1844*, trans. M. Milligan (New York: Prometheus Books).
—— (1990) *Capital: A Critique of Political Economy: Volume I*, trans. B. Fowkes (London: Penguin Books).
—— (2000) 'Theses on Feuerbach' in *Selected Writings*, ed. D. McLellan (Oxford: Oxford University Press).
Mazis, G.A. (2006) 'Facing Levinas: Merleau-Ponty's Physiognomic Ethics' in J. Hatley, J. McLane, C. Diehm (eds) *Interrogating Ethics: Embodying the Good in Merleau-Ponty* (Pittsburgh: Duquesne University Press).
McDonald, R. (2009) 'Preface' in S. Beckett, *Endgame* (London: Faber and Faber).
Menke, C. (2004) 'Genealogy and Critique: Two Forms of Ethical Questioning of Morality in T. Huhn (ed.) *The Cambridge Companion to Adorno* (Cambridge: Cambridge University Press).
—— (2006) *Reflections of Equality*, transl. H. Rouse, A. Denejkine (Stanford, CA: Stanford University Press).
Merleau-Ponty, M. (1958) *Phenomenology of Perception*, transl. C. Smith (London: Routledge).
—— (1964) 'The Primacy of Perception and Its Philosophical Consequences' in *The Primacy of Perception and Other Essays on Phenomenological Psychology, the*

Philosophy of Art, History and Politics, ed. J.M. Edie, transl. J.M. Edie (Evanston: Northwestern University Press).
—— (1968) *The Visible and the Invisible*, ed. Claude Lefort, transl. Alphonso Lingis (Evanston: Northwestern University Press).
—— (2004) *The World of Perception*, transl. O. Davis (London: Routledge).
Mishima, Y. (2003) *Sun and Steel*, transl. J. Bester (Tokyo: Kodansha International).
Müller-Doohm, S. (2003) *Adorno. Eine Biographie* (Frankfurt/M: Suhrkamp).
Muratori, C. (2008) 'Descartes. Error and the Barbarity of Western Philosophy. Schopenhauer in Dialogue with Coetzee's Elizabeth Costello', *Jahrbuch der Schopenhauer-Gesellschaft*, 89, 177–86.
New York Times (1987) 'Coetzee, Getting Prize, Denounces Apartheid', *The New York Times* (11 April 1987), nytimes.com, last visited: 31 May 2014, <http://www.nytimes.com/1987/04/11/arts/coetzee-getting-prize-denounces-apartheid.html>.
Nietzsche, F. (1974) *The Gay Science*, transl. W. Kauffmann (New York: Random House).
—— (1986) *The Anti-Christ*, transl. R.J. Hollingdale (London: Penguin Books).
—— (1997) *Daybreak: Thoughts on the Prejudices of Morality*, ed. M. Clark, B. Leiter, transl. R.J. Hollingdale (Cambridge: Cambridge University Press).
Nixon, M. (2011) *Samuel Beckett's German Diaries 1936–1937* (London: Continuum).
Nussbaum, M.C. (1999) 'Nietzsche, Schopenhauer, and Dionysus' in C. Janaway (ed.) *The Cambridge Companion to Schopenhauer* (Cambridge: Cambridge University Press).
Oppenheimer, J. (2012) *The Act of Killing* [DVD] (Copenhagen: Final Cut for Real).
Pessoa, F. (2006) *A Little Larger than the Entire Universe*, transl. ed. R. Zenith (London: Penguin Books).
Peters, M. (2013a) 'Will and Flesh: Schopenhauer and Merleau-Ponty on Corporeality', *Jahrbuch der Schopenhauer-Gesellschaft*, 94, 91–114.
—— (2013b) '"The Zone of the Carcass and the Knacker"—On Adorno's Concern with the Suffering Body', *European Journal of Philosophy*, doi: 10.1111/ejop.12048.
Proust, M. (1992) *In Search of Lost Time. Volume 1: Swann's Way*, transl. C.K.S. Moncrieff, T. Kilmartin (New York: Modern Library).
Raponi, S. (2003) 'Meaning and Melancholia in Beckett's Endgame', *Journal of Social and Political Thought*, 1(4), 1–22.
Raj Singh, R. (2007) *Death, Contemplation and Schopenhauer* (Hampshire: Ashgate).
Robertson, R. (2002) 'Kafka as Anti-Christian: "Das Urteil," "Die Verwandlung," and the Aphorisms' in J. Rolleston (ed.) *A companion to the Works of Franz Kafka* (Rochester, NY: Camden House).
—— (2004) *Kafka: A Very Short Introduction* (Oxford: Oxford University Press).
Rose, G. (1978) *The Melancholy Science: An Introduction to the Thought of Theodor W. Adorno* (London: Macmillan).
Rowles, D. (2014) 'Nic Pizzolatto Teases Season Two of "True Detective"', *Pajiba*. (10 March 2014), Pajiba.com, last visited 31 May 2014, <http://www.pajiba.com/trade_news/nic-pizzolatto-teases-season-two-of-true-detective.php>.

Ryan, M.P. (1999) 'Samsa and Samsara: Suffering, Death and Rebirth in the Metamorphosis', *German Quarterly*, 72, 113–52.
Sade, D.A.F. de (1965) *Justine: Or the Misfortunes of Virtue*, transl. A.H. Walton (London: Corgi Books).
Said, E. (2003) 'Dignity, Solidarity and the Penal Colony', *Counterpunch* (25 September 2003), Counterpunch.org, last visited: 31 May 2014, <http://www.counterpunch.org/2003/09/25/dignity-solidarity-and-the-penal-colony/>.
Sartre, J.P. (1984) *Being and Nothingness*, transl. H.E. Barnes (New York, NY: Washington Square Press).
Scarry, E. (1985) *The Body in Pain: The Making and Unmaking of the World* (New York: Oxford University Press).
Scheler, M. (1979) *The Nature of Sympathy*, transl. P. Heath (London: Routledge).
Schmicking, D. (2012) 'Schopenhauer und Merleau-Ponty – eine erste Annäherung' in M. Jeske, M. Koßler (eds) *Philosophie des Leibes. Die Anfänge bei Schopenhauer und Feuerbach* (Würzburg: Königshausen & Neumann).
Schmidt, A. (2004) 'Schopenhauer und der Materialismus' in *Tugend und Weltlauf. Vorträge und Aufsätze über die Philosophie Schopenhauers (1960–2003)* (Frankfurt am Main: Lang).
Schmied, W. (1996) *Francis Bacon: Commitment and Conflict*, transl. J. Ormrod (Munich: Prestel).
Schrödinger, E. (2001) *What is Life? With Mind and Matter & Autobiographical Sketches* (Cambridge: Cambridge University Press).
Schroeder, S. (2012) 'Schopenhauer's Influence on Wittgenstein' in B. Vandenabeele (ed.) *A Companion to Schopenhauer* (Oxford: Blackwell Publishing).
Schweppenhäuser G. (2004) 'Adorno's Negative Moral Philosophy' in T. Huhn (ed.) *The Cambridge Companion to Adorno* (Cambridge: Cambridge University Press).
Simmel, G. (1991) *Schopenhauer and Nietzsche*, transl. H. Loiskandl, D. Weinstein, M. Weinstein (Chicago, IL: University of Illinois Press).
Singer, P. (1999) 'Reflections' in J.M. Coetzee [et al] *The Lives of Animals*, ed. A. Gutman (Princeton, NJ: Princeton University Press).
Smith, A. (2007) *The Theory of Moral Sentiments* (Milton Keynes: Filiquarian Publishing).
Spierling, V. (1985) 'Erkenntnis und Ethik' in A. Schopenhauer, *Metaphysik der Sitten (Philosophische Vorlesungen, Teil IV)*, ed. V. Spierling (München: Piper Verlag).
Stokes, H.S. (1975) *The Life and Death of Yukio Mishima* (Tokyo: Charles E. Tuttle Company).
Swaab, D.F. (1014) *We are our Brains. A Neurobiography of the Brain: From the Womb to Alzheimer's*, transl. J. Hedley-Prôle (New York: Random House).
Tolstoy, L. (1965) *A Confession*, transl. J. Kentish (London: Penguin Books).
The Upanishads (1965) transl. J. Mascaró (London: Penguin Books).
Vandenabeele, B. (2009) 'Schopenhauer on Aesthetic Understanding and the Values of Art' in A. Neil, C. Janaway (eds) *Better Consciousness: Schopenhauer's Philosophy of Value* (Chisester: Wiley-Blackwell).
—— (2012) 'Introduction: Arthur Schopenhauer: The Man and His Work' in B. Vandenabeele (ed.) *A Companion to Schopenhauer* (Oxford: Blackwell Publishing).

Vandenrath, J. (1977) 'Pessimismus und Marxismus, *Jahrbuch der Schopenhauer-Gesellschaft*, 58, 15–29.
Veauthier, F.W. (1988) 'Zur Transformation der Pessimismus – Motive im Denken Max Horkheimers', *Jahrbuch der Schopenhauer-Gesellschaft*, 69, 593–607.
Vetlesen, A.J. (2009) *A Philosophy of Pain*, transl. J. Irons (London: Reaktion Books).
Voltaire (2006) *Candide and Other Stories*, transl. R. Pearson (Oxford: Oxford University Press).
de Waal, F. (2006) *Primates and Philosophers: How Morality Evolved*, ed. S. Macedo, J. Ober (Princeton: Princeton University Press).
—— (2009) *The Age of Empathy: Nature's Lessons for a Kinder Society* (New York: Harmony Books).
White, F.C. (1999) 'The Fourfold Root' in C. Janaway (ed.) *The Cambridge Companion to Schopenhauer* (Cambridge: Cambridge University Press).
Whitebook, J. (2004) 'Weighty Objects: On Adorno's Kant-Freud Interpretation' in T. Huhn (ed.) *The Cambridge Companion to Adorno* (Cambridge: Cambridge University Press).
Wicks, R. (2012) 'Schopenhauer's On the Will in Nature: The Reciprocal Containment of Idealism and Realism' in B. Vandenabeele (ed.) *A Companion to Schopenhauer* (Oxford: Blackwell Publishing).
Wilde, O. (1954) *De Profundis and Other Writings* (Harmondsworth: Penguin Books).
Wischke, M. (1994) *Die Geburt der Ethik: Schopenhauer – Nietzsche – Adorno* (Berlin: Akademie Verlag).
—— (1996) 'Nähe und Differenz in der Moralphilosophie von A. Schopenhauer und Th. W. Adorno', *Jahrbuch der Schopenhauer-Gesellschaft*, 77, 181–97.
Wittgenstein L. (1958) *Philosophical Investigations*, transl. G.E.M. Anscombe (Oxford: Basil Blackwell).
—— (2001) *Tractatus Logico-Philosophicus*, transl. D.F. Pears, B.F. McGuinness (London: Routledge).
Young, J. (1987) *Willing and Unwilling: A Study in the Philosophy of Arthur Schopenhauer* (Dordrecht: Martinus Nijhoff Publishers).
—— (1988) 'Is Schopenhauer an Irrationalist?', *Jahrbuch der Schopenhauer-Gesellschaft*, 69, 85–100.
—— (2009) 'Schopenhauer, Nietzsche, Death and Salvation' in A. Neil, C. Janaway (eds) *Better Consciousness: Schopenhauer's Philosophy of Value* (Chisester: Wiley-Blackwell).
Zaretsky, E. (2005) *Secrets of the Soul: A Social and Cultural History of Psychoanalysis* (New York: Vintage Books).
Zenith, R. (2006) 'Introduction: The Birth of a Nation' in F. Pessoa, *A Little Larger than the Entire Universe*, transl., ed. R. Zenith (London: Penguin Books).
Zilcosky, J. (2007) 'Kafka Approaches Schopenhauer's Castle', *German Life and Letters*, 44, 353–69.
Zuidervaart, L. (1991) *Adorno's Aesthetic Theory: The Redemption of Illusion* (Cambridge, MA: The MIT Press).
—— (2007) *Social Philosophy after Adorno* (Cambridge: Cambridge University Press).

Index

9781137412164